THE MAKING OF LETTERS TO DANIEL

AMY MCCORKLE

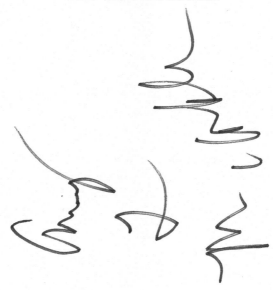

ERUDITE PRESS

ISBN: 978-1-937979-97-3

Erudite Press

Goshen, Kentucky 40026

www.eruditepress.com

INTRODUCTION

I was privileged to view the debut of Amy Leigh McCorkle's film, *Letters to Daniel*. When Tony Acree asked me to edit this book about the making of the movie, it did not take me long to fall in love with both the story, and the concept.

When I met Amy at the 2019 Imaginarium Convention, she told me that her film would be debuting the next day, Saturday, October 12, so I made it a point to attend. Minutes before the screening, I took my seat and waited, with the rest of the audience, for the movie to begin.

The cast did a good job portraying the friendship, and raw emotion, between Amy and Missy. It's amazing all that Amy underwent during the making of her award-winning film. My words cannot even attempt to do it justice, so you will just have to read all about it, right here, for yourselves.

Millions of people worldwide suffer from bipolar disorder. It is an emotionally crippling disease which affects much more than a person's mental state of being. Because of that, many have a difficult time controlling their emotions. Sometimes, sadly, people who are diagnosed with the disease get mislabeled as "crazy people," which is not the case at all.

One of the key points of *Letters to Daniel* is to raise awareness about bipolar disorder, and let the audience know that those who suffer from it need are no different from the rest of us. Because of Amy's perseverance, and her strong bond with Missy, she is able to fight back against the disease and live out God's plan for her life.

Writing letters to celebrities can sometimes be cathartic, which only makes sense because Daniel Craig is Amy's favorite actor. What started out as a simple letter went on to become a blog, then a film, which includes the interest and talents of many.

And, while Amy has yet to meet Daniel in person, she enjoyed the experience of writing to him. As a result, her work was fueled by hope, and she made many new friends along the journey of making the film.

Excitement rushed through my veins during the awards ceremony, especially since *Recovery Unplugged* was up for Best Independent Screenplay; it received runner up.

A few moments later, I heard my own name being called. *You Are You!* had just won the IMADJINN Award for 2019 Best Children's Book. Needless to say, I was elated, and part of the reason for that was because my work was honored the same night as Amy.

After the ceremony, Amy and I congratulated each other on our victories. Her happiness was contagious, as everyone else at the banquet seemed to share in her delight. That had not been the first time her work won any accolades, or awards, so I know that this is just one of many great achievements that Amy will have during her lifetime.

--Jen Selinsky, October 2019

A JOURNEY OF A THOUSAND MILES

*I*t all started seven years ago, when I had a conversation with my first publisher, MuseItUP in Canada, owned by Lea Schizas. I had recently done well with blog about writing, as I stacked awards interactions on my blog along the way. However, in January of 2012, I had one published book, with another two coming out. And, by that point, *everyone* had a blog about writing, which led to the afore-mentioned conversation. Now that I've done the pre-requisite blog about writing, where do I go from here, as far as platform and brand building?

Lea planted this seed: *Why don't you get some other writers with bipolar disorder and do a blog about that?*

I promptly dismissed that idea. Getting together a group of writers with the same disease as I had, to write in an orderly fashion, would be akin to herding to cats. I didn't give it another thought. I toured with my books to conventions and bookstores, and simply became a writing machine.

Since 2011, I have penned thirty books, twenty-four which

have been published. So, really, you could say that it goes back to 2009, when I rented *Casino Royale* and became hooked on all things starring Daniel Craig.

He became the template for all the heroes whom I would write about. Whether it be a hybrid human-alien, a mercenary, a struggling addict, striving to better himself through his music, or a cleaner falling in love with his mark.

In 2012, I began writing screenplays again. Using my books, I would adapt the material and I would "cast" Daniel in the starring male roles. Currently, I am co-writing my thirty-third screenplay with Melissa Goodman.

We have known each other and written together for over twenty years. In 2012, we adapted my bestselling novel, *Bounty Hunter*, to script form.

Then, in 2013, an odd thing happened. I decided to write Daniel Craig an open letter, in the form of a blogpost, and I named the blog *Letters to Daniel*. About halfway through the letter, (post) I realized that I was trying to squeeze in a lifetime of experiences, and his work's enormous impact on my career, and recovery, that I wouldn't be able to write just one letter encompassing my whole lifetime.

The first letter of the blog gives the general context, but it's wholly unlike the rest of the blog. I decided to use the letters as a way of telling my life story, present and future. It was a way to process my illness, and I believe it became a piece of my healing, and recovery, regarding bipolar disorder. Daniel inspired me but, the way that I wrote to him, it could have been anybody. Dear God, or Dear Diary, would have same effect, but for having Daniel there as a sort of silent, non-judgmental witness to my daily pain made me less self-conscious about revealing the true parts of myself, without worrying about what other people would think of me, and without worrying who would be mad at me.

It was my life. Figuring that Daniel Craig didn't have a social media footprint, there was a certain anonymity to what I was doing. What I didn't expect was the response that I would receive from some of my readers, such as, *"There was a lot of good information on here, I feel you are telling my story,"* or, *"Thank you for this, my daughter has bipolar disorder."*

By October of 2013, I had amassed enough letters to put together a thin volume. I self-published it on Amazon, where it hit #2 in autobiographies.

In February of 2014, I published a second volume of the letters. I just had burning desire to tell my story, as well as to help others who are struggling with bipolar disorder.

I wasn't finished conquering my demons; those never really go away. I was more than driven to take the next step forward, so I contacted Stephen Zimmer. He was planning the inaugural year of Imaginarium, and he wanted to have a film festival. I asked him if there would be a category for documentaries.

He said that there would be. When I told about the idea for my documentary, he gave me a premiere, and a Q&A panel. I didn't even have a documentary finished yet!

That documentary cost me $345 to make, including the entry fees. That was during the spring of 2014. That zero-budget proof of concept doc travelled well on the circuit and inspired both me and Missy to adapt my memoir to a narrative script about how we survived poverty, stigma, mental illness, loss, and one another. It proceeded to be selected, nominated, and won second place and Most Original Screenplay across several festivals.

We then set about shopping the script to independent

producers. Each of them pretty much said, "I don't have the resources," or "I don't have the time."

It was mine and Missy's second year at Indie Gathering, and we had won ten awards there. It was amazing to walk up to the front that many times. I sat down with a filmmaking team there and pitched *Letters to Daniel* to them. I said, "Come on board," and they said, "Yes."

What followed was me doing all the work, and growing increasingly manic, while my other producers in New York did nothing.

When we were nine days out from the shoot, with the cast locked in, and the locations secured, these people had an argument, and they brought it to my front door, in the form of Facebook messages, at 2:00 in the morning. One of them was freaking out and demanded that I do something about a situation which they had discussed with the other half of the team.

I reached out, repeatedly, to his partner on FB, and by phone, and all I got was radio silence. At that point, I realized that they were forcing my hand. If I had proceeded with production, it would have, most likely, been an unmitigated disaster. They shit all over my dream and, in turn, devastated me. I was forced to pull the plug.

I had to call a casting director, who had worked for free, and inform her about what happened. I also had to tell the cast. In fact, I had to call all the locations and notify them. My recovery was set so far back that I ran, head long, into a toxic manager/client relationship.

They said things like, "Just because I award your script doesn't mean that it's any good. Pam, you're a great writer. Amy, you're okay." They were trying to get me to sell *Letters to Daniel* for less than what it was worth, all the while constantly trying to separate me from Missy. And, when they said, "You don't look like you have a disability," and "You don't act like you have a disability." I knew that I had to part company with them. But they would dig in their claws and leave me vulnerable. They were shady, at best, and I wasn't their only victim. However, they threatened on my way out the door, but I finally gathered up the nerve to say no to them. Then, I took my work and moved on.

Unfortunately, I left them for an unstable, unwell, and unreliable woman who lied about funding $20,000 for my movie. (It never materialized.) She also lied about a company offering me a publishing contract for me for my novel.

Even though I learned a lot about running a set and directing. *Black Gold: The Trail to Standing Rock* was one of the worst experiences I'd ever had on set. My crew didn't listen to me; they held my movie hostage, and they only took orders from the aforementioned woman.

It was a steep learning curve. That woman did do one service, however; she encouraged me to go all in at the 2016 Action On Film International Film Festival. I got in five scripts and three film projects.

I only found out the festival date two months prior. Now, if you know anything about me, you know that, as of this time of writing, I am currently on disability, and I take in $779.00 a month. I did a GoFundMe fundraiser and raised enough for the hotel. Through more donations, I had accumulated $385, which my food budget for ten days in Monrovia, CA.

God Bless my Aunt Sue, even though she pisses me off massively sometimes. She let me tag along with her as she drove out to visit her daughter in San Diego. Aunt Sue also paid for all the gas, and the hotel rooms, during the six-day journey, both there and back.

My first year at AOF was mind-blowing, life-changing, and

career-altering. It was my first west coast festival, and my itty-bitty proof that *Letters to Daniel* was nominated for Best Social Commentary, as well as the Louis Mitchell Award for Best Feature, or Short.

Not only that, but Missy and myself were nominated for Best SciFi/Fantasy Script in Bounty Hunter, Best Short Scene in Back On Top, and Best New Writers at AOF.

There were over 20,000 people in attendance: filmmakers, screenwriters, composers, and artists from all across the globe. Del and Theresa were warm, and welcoming. Theresa is a beast at running the festival. Del is a creative genius who is both brilliant, and charismatic.

That first year, I was a fish out of water, yet everyone there embraced me as an equal. Del and Theresa showered me (like they do all their creators) with unconditional love, acceptance, and encouragement. Del had also taken me under his wing and mentored me.

That first year, I would meet two people who would become fixtures in my creative life, Clint Gaige; (*A Clean Exit, Fat Guy w/ a Shotgun 1 & 2,* and *Hell Is Empty*) he has become a mentor, and a creative collaborator. And Mark Maness has become a mentor, friend, and collaborator. We were all a part of the AOF Class of 2016.

Over the years, I would make documentaries and short films, gaining experience and feedback from these individuals. Thomas Moore was an ally as well because he struggled with mental illness, like me. He's also an uber talented filmmaker.

The final piece of my dream team crew was Valyo Gennoff, a sound editor and composer. His music raises the level of all my projects. And I can't wait for him to score *Letters to Daniel*.

In 2017, I had a pitch package put together. With the rest of my dream team coming about: from Film-Com, my 1AD

Abigail Yates, from Indie Gathering, my Script Supervisor Doug Kaufman, my Producer, extraordinaire Missy Goodman, on sound, Justin Simmons and Jules Leskiv, on slate, whoever picked up. These people, along with talented cast, put their faith in me and, together, we would go on an incredible adventure.

2

DEL AND THERESA WESTON: LIFE CHANGERS, GAME CHANGERS

2016 was a tumultuous year for me. There was the good: mine and *Missy's Letters to Daniel* script being nominated at the International Christian Film Festival, NOVA, and the Los Angeles Independent Film Awards. The eight project acceptance into Action On Film, and subsequent wins at LAIFA, and AOF.

The bad: My mental health had been majorly compromised by the actions of the flaky filmmakers who had forced the first pushback of *Letters to Daniel*. I'd been sent into a downward spiral and, as a result, this left me vulnerable to some predatory players on the local scene, ones who had a reputation for being shady at best, downright evil, at worst.

At the time, in early 2016, I had accomplished something amazing. *Letters to Daniel* was on the paid bestsellers list on Amazon, and those people wanted a part that. Needless to say, I got entangled with them and had a hell of a time extracting myself from the situation, but I did and, within a few months, I had entered AOF.

Let me explain something here. I called AOF, and Del Weston answered. First, let be said that, in a world full of imitators, Del is the genuine article. Big, bold, brash, and charismatic Del is a genius, and a brilliant light shining on hill, guiding creators, near and far, to join the AOF family and benefit from this unique event.

My first impression of Del was one of overwhelming warmth and enthusiasm. I told him about my projects, and he wanted to see them all. He ended his sentences with, "Yeah, baby," and it didn't come off as put on, or fake. For the record, Del Weston doesn't have a fake bone in his body.

So I entered what I felt were the best of the best that Missy and me had to offer. Then, I promptly let it go. When I checked out the official AOF website, it was huge. *There's no way I'm getting in,* I thought.

I went about the business of writing my next novel. My first 70K novel, as a matter of fact. And the book, itself, fought me tooth and nail to be written, so that kept me occupied. About halfway through June, I received notification that I had indeed been selected for AOF.

As excited as I was, I faced several obstacles in getting there. The first one being, how was I going to get there? The second, where was I going to get the money? And, third, how would I eat, and get around in Monrovia, CA, a place I didn't know anything about?

The fact was that I had to get there. In fact, Del teased me in front of an audience, and said I called him no less than thirty-two times, saying, "I don't know how I going to do it, but I'm going to get there."

As I have mentioned before, my aunt was going out west, and she allowed me to tag along. Of course, I had to endure her history lessons, and whacked out political talk but, in the long

9

run, it was worth it. Just, after six days in a car with her, I was ready for the adventure to be over.

For the rest of the money, I did a GoFundMe. I raised $700. That, with my disability check, got me my hotel room, and $385 left to eat on.

Although I talked big on social media about going to California for AOF, inside, I was totally intimidated.

The first person to greet me upon arrival was the amazing Harold L. Brown. He told me, at first, that he didn't like the way I was on social media. He then continued to say that I grew on him, and that he changed his mind about me. I had to laugh. Harold is the sweetest man, so giving of his time and expertise, always there for friends when they need him. Not only that, but he is one of the most gifted writers whom I have ever met.

I checked in and met Susana Compos and Christine Whalen. Susana would save me when my blood sugar bottomed out; she got me a large popcorn and a soda.

Finally, I spied Del setting up the drop banner, and the red carpet, so that people could take pictures and promote their films.

He caught sight of me and broke out into a huge smile. He then called me over and gave me a bear hug, saying that he was excited to see me. To catch a wave of love that big right off the bat was huge, but it also threw me for a loop. No other festival had been that effusive.

He had Ron Podell take me to dinner, along with another festival attendee. I forget his name but, when I returned to the theater, where the hub of activity was and saw Harold again, he sat down and excitedly told me that he had been doing some writing and met up with a big name Canadian actor who wanted to team up with him. Harold has always been generous with his time, and his wisdom. Harold was patient with the jittery, anxious, and a just happy to be invited to the party screenwriter and filmmaker in me.

I was supposed to be at the dinner w/Del that year, but my documentary was screening at the same time, so I skipped the dinner and went to my film's screening. Fortunately, as I had very little money, many guardian angels stepped in and fed me during the week.

A filmmaker whom I had met briefly in the corridors was Clint Gaige, West Virginian filmmaker whose project that year was *A Clean Exit*. He was friendly and said, "I'm sorry that I couldn't make your film's screening, but I believe in what you're doing."

I watched him win at the awards dinner, and he was as humble as he was talented. I promptly added him as Facebook friend and began building a mentor/protégé relationship with him.

Another filmmaker I met there is Arkansas native, Mark Maness, director of *It Knows*, and *Birthrite*, among others. His cinematography talents are indescribable. I wanted both of those men on my team. I befriended Mark and spent some more time with him over the course of the week, and I added him as a FB friend, too.

Those two would become two of my biggest cheerleaders, and advisors, and the only reason I found them was because I had been welcomed into the AOF fold. Del Weston said the point of AOF is for creators to network, work together, and create little AOF babies together.

Theresa, when I was disconnected from everybody, encouraged me to come to the charity Paint N' Play, where at risk kids completed a charity project and enjoyed refreshments. I met Matt Sconce there. It's funny when lives touch. He recently went public on FB with his bipolar 2 diagnosis. He's a massively talented director, and writer and, now, role-playing game inventor. He also creates DCP's for AOFers. And that is yet another way AOF has upped my game as a filmmaker.

By that point, I was waiting for the miracle twenty grand to materialize so that I could make my dream project, *Letters to Daniel*. But AOF was giving me the tools to create my own little miracle, I just didn't know it yet.

Finally, I took Del's seminar, Del Weston's *Get It Done*.

What that man knows about the film industry, along with the oodles of talent that he possesses, made the seminar a must attend. What I would find out during those two hours was that one, Del was as gifted teaching the craft as he was at executing it, two, that he had a passion to guide others to their dreams, and three, he had a bullshit detector set at a low threshold. Also, if he decided to take you under his wing, then he saw something special in you, even if you didn't notice it yet.

I was so fired up and inspired that I went home, cast *Broken*, and made plans to direct it, with Missy producing. I made *Black Gold* that winter. *Broken* was Heaven. *Black Gold* was Hell.

If the 2016 Action On Film taught me anything, it's that no one was going to make your debut film for you; you had go out there and do it yourself.

The awards ceremonies, one for written word, and one for film and video, were watershed events for both me and Missy. Even though Missy was not in attendance, her presence was very much felt. When our names were announced for Best New Writer at AOF, I struggled to keep my composure, and hold back my tears, as I thanked AOF, and all the attendees, for what they had done for me over the previous ten days. And what that was, they renewed my belief that *Letters to Daniel* could be made, that I could direct it, and that me and Missy had a chance of launching up to the next level. All of it was within my grasp, I just had to step out on faith and put action behind it.

At the film and video awards show, I would take home Best Social Commentary. Holding back powerful emotions I don't remember a word I said. Standing before so many people, beating out films that I felt were far superior to mine, all that was all a blur.

The Queen of AOF, Anabelle Munro, said that I gave an eloquent speech in which I talked about bipolar disorder and wanted to help others with it. I remember thanking Missy's father, who had died six years prior, and that's about all.

I try not to write acceptance speeches, as I feel they are jinxes. I suppose that I'm superstitious, at least when it comes to that.

Del and Theresa have become constant supporters of mine and Missy's work. They were the first ones who really pushed me to direct, even when I was facing doubters, and setbacks (besides Missy). I love Del and Theresa. AOF 2016 changed my life and forever altered the direction of my career in the film industry. They renewed my fighting spirits. And, throughout the years, I have healed, due in no small part to AOF, *Letters to Daniel* is finally a reality.

3

RAY SZUCH AND KRISTINA MICHELLE: VALIDATORS, CHEERLEADERS

*I*n 2014, I made a proof of concept documentary, *Letters to Daniel: Breakdown to Bestseller*. I took a selection of the letters, the greatest hits, if you will, and formed a narrative. I then placed a selection of still photographs over and provided my own voice-over for the project. I entered it into Imaginarium Film Festival because I had been invited to.

I got a Withoutabox (a soon to be defunct film submission platform) email screaming about a May 15th deadline for a film festival which I had submitted four screenplays to already. Completely on a lark, I decided to enter my little film to this festival called Indie Gathering.

Understand that the talent they pull to their small festival is incredible. I had no way of knowing that at the time. My scripts did well there, but my films were the Honorable Mention also rans of the festival. No matter how I tried to improve, it had been the same.

That being said, there were plenty of entrants that didn't get HM. They were simply not included in the festival. But, for my first documentary, *Letters to Daniel: Breakdown to Bestseller,* I didn't expect anything.

And honorable mention is an amazing thing at Indie Gathering, you have to score at least 90 percent out of 100 percent to get an honorable mention, so it's like your film getting the grade of B+.

In 2014, I didn't consider myself a filmmaker. Even though I had done the documentary, I primarily saw myself as a screenwriter, and an author. So when *Letters to Daniel* was given an Honorable Mention that first year, I was thrilled beyond belief. As much as I had enjoyed making the documentary, I didn't think that it had much artistic, or technical, merit.

Ray is an exception to this, he takes pride in his film festival. He says, if you get an award there, that you earned it. I've had twenty-two film projects there, two second places, a 3rd place, and a 4th place. Second places were a microfilm and a proof of concept trailer. Any complete film has not risen above 3rd. I'll be honest that, with *Letters to Daniel,* I hoped to take home 1st place. But the competition was fierce, and Indie Gathering has gained a reputation (rightfully so) as a festival that highly regards talent.

I'm just a competitive little shit, and having a string of honorable mention means I'm not taking enough risks, and I'm not delivering as great a product as I want. I set out to change that with mine and Missy's *Letters to Daniel* feature film.

We'll see how it turns out. As of now, I will be looking at a cut of the film next Friday. Being able to enter it into festivals will be nice, but I had so wished it would have been longer.

Anyway, Ray and Kristina's festival planted the seed in my head that my dream of directing could, indeed, happen, just on a different level. I didn't want a different level. Meaning, I would have to find people who would work for free, pay them in gas, IMDb food and, in some cases, shelter.

I wanted some bankroll for me. But the truth is that no wants to bankroll someone else's dream, especially a film. They're risky as hell, and there's never any real guarantee that they're going to pay off, at least with an independent film, that is.

With *Letters to Daniel*, I wanted to leap to the next level, career wise. As filled with sharks and ne'er do and predators as it is, we want Hollywood success. But I suppose that everyone does.

In 2015, Missy and I co-wrote the screenplay for *Letters to Daniel*, and we achieved, you guessed it, honorable mention. In 2018, we would revise the script and re-enter it; we still couldn't shake the honorable mention label.

Other places it would be nominated and selected were at the NOVA, where it won the Jury Award, at LAIFFA, it took home 2nd Place and, at Script Summit, it would win Most Original Screenplay.

That being said, Ray and Kristina, like Del and Theresa, really believed in what me and Missy were doing with the *Letters to Daniel* project. They were always there, cajoling, encouraging, and giving us a platform to push the brand out into the ethers, as it were.

I initially attended Indie Gathering in 2014 with my Aunt Sue. Missy wouldn't take off for it. We would win five awards. It marked the first time that a for real, legit film festival was honoring our work, and that was huge.

Sometimes, I have to go before Missy will. I am truly a Gemini, and she is truly a Taurus. She doesn't trust easily and, if she doesn't trust you, she'll shake you until your break. Whereas, I am, perhaps, a little too quick to trust. We complimented each other nicely and, the next year, Missy would attend and, once again, we would establish ourselves, at least, as solid writers by winning ten awards.

To date, we have submitted fifty-nine projects to the Indie Gathering and won fifty-seven. Some would say that we have nothing to prove.

Until now, it has been enough to hit the board. Missy and I were at a point where we wanted the championship belt, either for the screenplay, of for the film. It doesn't really matter which one, we just covet it.

Back to 2018, we attended the Indie Gathering and went and watched a short film by William Johns, in the hope of wooing him to produce *Letters to Daniel*.

Peter John Ross and William joined me and Missy afterwards for a drink (I bought a round) and pitched *Letters to Daniel* to William.

William begged off and volunteered Ross.

Ross, in turn, suggested an Aaron Allen from the Cincinnati area.

I friended him on FB and, within the week, *Letters to Daniel* had an executive producer who would work hard in finding us money for the film.

Indie Gathering was where we'd find a lot of our team. Doug Kaufman, a fixture at Horror Hotel, and semi-regular at Indie Gathering, became our script supervisor, and he really shined in pre-production by taking a lot of pressure off of me. I met Brandon X Bell there in 2016 and, through him, I would connect with Laura Masi Cline, and her son, Michael, as well as John Spalding of G1NBC (more about him later). I would then also connect with Valyo Gennoff, a soft spoken, and modest, but an immensely talented composer. (More on Doug, Brandon, John, and Valyo later.)

The magic of Indie Gathering is the array of talent they pool there and how many amazing connections result in collaborative art. Independent film.

Networking is what Ray is all about. He will pull you into conversations with would be producers, connect you with directors, actors and, in my case, multiple composers.

Famously, last year, Ray kind of pushed a composer upon me, and I did NOT want to sit down and talk to him. I had my composer. I had no need for music. Yet, as I spoke to Ricardo Raymundo, he asked me what I wanted. I said that I wanted a song written specifically for the end credits of *Letters to Daniel*.

He then said that he and his daughter would come up with something.

I sent them the script, told them what I was looking for, and checked in with him in December.

At the end of February, he messaged me, saying that, within few weeks, I'd have the song, and he'd go on to tell me why this song was so important to both him and his daughter.

Finally, a month later, I received an email with the song attached. It was the most beautiful thing I'd ever heard, and it fit perfectly with the movie.

Ricardo went on to explain that his daughter, the singer/songwriter of the song, "Here with Me," had been something of a rising star. She sang for theater and film, done voice work for Disney, and even had some traction on her music. Then, his younger son was diagnosed with Leukemia, and depression hit her hard. She quit everything. No warning, no tapering off, no nothing.

Then, I requested a song for *Letters to Daniel*. It was the first thing she had written and performed since her brother's diagnosis.

Warner Music heard and first offered her a distribution

deal, using *Letters to Daniel*'s logo as packaging, and then extended it to an artist's contract. The collaboration had truly resulted in a beautiful thing, and it would not have happened were it not for Ray Szuch forcing me to talk to Ricardo at Indie Gathering. I will be forever indebted to Ray for that.

Indie Gathering is a beautiful place, where beautiful things happen. I was unable to attend during 2019, due to financial reasons. But, I will be back, with a ton of scripts, and *Letters to Daniel*, in tow.

Indie Gathering, while not presenting me with large opportunities, they have given me the tools I need to capitalize on those large opportunities when they present themselves.

Indie Gathering has allowed me to network with a team of people whom I can regularly depend on in order to execute any of my films. And it does so while remaining relatively affordable to the independent filmmaker, which all know is dependent upon the kindness of strangers, and their friends and families, to get anything down.

I usually have three festivals that I attend every year. But, for that year, I had to sit out my Ohio home away from home. Missy couldn't afford it. And our friend, Pam, who usually comes with us was facing her home front battles.

Suffice to say, were it not for Indie Gathering validating our work, and teaching us about the power of networking, *Letters to Daniel* may still just a blog, a popular blog. I needed blog, a healing blog, but it would be a project whose potential was pretty much unrealized.

4

STEPHEN ZIMMER AND THE IMAGINARIUM

*S*tephen Zimmer is a prolific independent author, director of the television pilot, *Rayden Valkryrie*, and creator and director of Imaginarium, a yearly creative writing convention which takes place in Louisville, KY around the first, or the second, weekend of October each year.

I got connected with Stephen, by chance in 2011, when I asked if I could be on panels at Fandom Fest. The 2011 edition was notoriously known as Sweat Fest. Seeing that the a/c had failed in the host hotel, and the vendors were all crammed into the center elbow, it was like going to your shady uncle's house whom you know was going to creep up on you.

That being said, two good things came out of that encounter, I met Stephen, and another author, Maurice Broaddus. (Another psychological sibling.)

Fandom Fest was, is, and always will be, shady. But, in 2013, Imaginarium was born, and Stephen Zimmer invited me to attend as a guest author. He mentioned that there would be a small film festival attached, but no screenplay contest that year.

The wheels in my head started turning. I envisioned a documentary about my struggles with bipolar disorder, but I couldn't get anyone to sit down with me and do an interview. Still, I very much wanted to direct a film about it.

So I approached Stephen and asked if there was a category for documentaries, and he said, "Yes."

I then told him my idea for the film.

He said, "Great we'll premiere it here, and you can do a Q&A."

I was high, for sure, but the only two films I had directed during my twenties were crap. That really didn't stop me, however. What I did, because my vision was totally coming together, was adapt.

A festival had invited me to attend, so I figured that I might as well make the most of it, and make a film. I selected a small group of letters, twelve or thirteen of what you would call the greatest hits so that it would form an impactful narrative. I also laid a series of photographs of me from the time when I was a baby, until I was at events, selling my novels.

I had enough titles that I got a vendor table at Imaginarium for me, Missy, Pam and, for that first year, my much younger cousin, Rebekah. I would sell thirty books, sit on panels, and screen my documentary.

When I arrived at Imaginarium that first year, I was humming with anticipation. It was the first year of the con and, though much smaller than any of the other events I would eventually go to, that year gave me lots of friends and supporters, who were also attending and selling their own books there.

As people walked around and decided whether or not to buy my books, I chatted them up. And, if they didn't purchase anything, then I highly encouraged them to come to the film.

My fur baby, Chyna, had lived for fourteen years and saw

me break through at the 2014 Indie Gathering. Chyna was an orange tabby who was borderline feral, yet I was her person. She tended to hiss at Missy (One time, Missy did throw a shoe at her, and it hit her, though). Chyna slept on my shoulder, my lap, and was always by my side when I would be working on a project.

Though she did live to see my big night at Imaginarium, she present on my McCorklefest T-Shirt.

Stephen, though not as big a presence as, say, Del or Ray, was the person who gave me a proverbial seat at the table, locally, because he accepted me; other writers deemed me worthy of hanging around with.

And, through the Kentuckiana Authors Fair, Conglomeration, Fandom Fest, and Imaginarium, the first four years of my professional development were pretty much successful, but uneventful.

I would be published through MuseItUP, Hydra, and Blackwyrm during those years. Eventually, I would branch out as an independent publisher. Going from one book to twenty-four, with eleven of those being Amazon Bestsellers.

As much as Daniel was actual inspiration for the art, and my staying in treatment, without Stephen Zimmer's generosity, I would have never had the access to the publishing companies, the authors, or just some of the really cool people I would meet, many of whom lived in the North Central Kentucky/Southern Indiana area.

You can throw a rock around here, and you hit a publishing house. But, if you don't know about them, how are you supposed to pitch them? My first three contracts came though a Canadian epublisher, MuseItUp Publishing, the same one responsible for putting a bug in my ear about the blog.

Stephen is the kind of guy who will sit down with new

writers and let them pick his brain for lessons to apply to their craft.

The first year of Imaginarium was one of my favorite convention experiences. I found out what it is to screen your hard, as I fought for work in front of a home crowd. I got to do a Q&A for the first time, and I sold a ton of books. It also didn't hurt that I was a runner up in the documentary category.

That being said, I think one of the most memorable things about that first Imaginarium was the fact someone pulled the fire alarm right out of the gate during first panels on the first day of the convention.

Stephen owns Seventh Star Press, Seventh Star Studios, and has a podcast, *The Star Chamber*. Like all independent artists, he far from wealthy, but he is generous with his time, his talent, and his heart.

He had quite the journey to his pilot, *Rayden*, made. It is based on a series of novels, and novellas (personally, I think they're his best) and, when it comes to your brain babies, you want to spend time with them and love them as much as possible.

William Goldman would say that's the whore talking. But, as you can see, *Letters to Daniel* has been many things, and it has served as a way for me to heal and advocate. And, when ideas strike, I feel like I'm dying to unload the experience.

When I directed *Black Gold: The Trail to Standing Rock*, it was a traumatic experience. My crew didn't listen to me, and we turned on one another. We produced a good film, but I could have edited the doc as well as anybody else, but I digress.

Stephen Zimmer's goal upon meeting any writer is to make them feel welcome. And he has built a charming, offbeat convention for people to gather and celebrate writing. *Letters to*

Daniel truly spent some of its formative incubation time at Imaginarium.

During the spring of 2016, Missy and I shot (with the assistance of good friend and author/screenwriter/director, Pamela Turner) the microfilm *Letters to Daniel: Awareness.* With Kat Salim as Amy, and Kelsey Walsh as Missy. They did a wonderful job, and it screened at Imaginarium in 2016, where it won Best Short Film.

When I needed a projector for the scene in the opening and closing sequences, Stephen and Holly Phillipe (Holly being Stephen's girlfriend and partner in business matters) rose to occasion. Got up at 4:15 in the more on the second day and came to the set, and he fully participated.

Stephen and Holly were truly angels for helping make my dream come true.

I had launched a novel and how-to book at Imaginarium in 2019, *The Guardian* and *Something to Believe In.*

Not only that, Stephen continues to support my mental health advocacy mission with *Letters to Daniel*, as well as subsequent works.

I will be teaching the workshop How to Thrive Creatively While Coping with Serious Mental Illness. I've never taught a workshop before, and this will be my first time out. It only seems appropriate that it's with Imaginarium.

I mentioned 2016 briefly. I should also say who has, without a doubt, become a good friend, and someone's whose opinions on filmmaking I find invaluable; fellow filmmaker, Thomas Moore. I would meet him while doing a documentary panel that year.

I would learn that he, too, struggles with bipolar disorder. So, besides being a filmmaker, there's that. I would watch his movies (he's got a great team around him) and marvel at his

24

technical achievements. Through him, I would meet actresses Megan Jones, and Virginia Beld.

Those two undiscovered powerhouses would give me their all on the set and then some.

Many people are fixtures at Imaginarium, such as super publisher/author/screenwriter/producer, Tony Acree. Be on the lookout for his movie adaptation of the *Hand of God*. He is amazing. He is also AARP Batman on Masquerade Ball night.

He is someone I admire, and even envy a little. But I don't begrudge him his success, not even for one minute. He's earned every last bit of it, and I couldn't be happier for him.

What I want people to know about Imaginarium is that it's a wonderful local convention, and it's a great place if you're just getting started in the creative industry. Not only that but, compared to many other cons, it's surprisingly affordable, and in a semi-decent hotel.

I, for one, will be staying there. As Imaginarium 2019 drew closer, I looked forward to *Letters to Daniel* test screening there. With Imaginarium heavily involved, my good friend (and best-selling author) Mysti Parker, saved my ass by providing her beautiful home as a location for us to use when someone else got cold feet.

Stephen Zimmer was the first professional writer and film-maker to say, "Welcome to the club. Take a seat, have a drink, and get to know everyone because everyone wants to get to know you."

Imaginarium is a lot like that as well. They favor sci-fi/fantasy/and horror films, and scripts, but there's plenty of room for other genres to come and play, too.

Imaginarium will always hold a special place in my heart, as will the *Letters to Daniel* documentary, because they both gave me two dear friends in Andrew and James. They no longer attend Imaginarium, as they're all the way out in California. But it's safe to say that, if Imaginarium had not screened *Letters to Daniel*, the documentary, Missy and me might have never written the script, and I certainly wouldn't have written this book.

5

VALYO GENNOFF: FIRST ONE ON BOARD

$\mathcal{U}$p until the 2016 film festival season, my documentaries either had no music, or music by Frozen Creek Studios. However, while their music was lovely, I needed to branch out and be more than a Stephen Zimmer sycophant. Even he wouldn't have me to do that.

Over the years, at Indie Gathering, Ray Szuch introduced me to countless composers. He always said, "See, Amy."

Sometimes, I would humor him, but I really didn't take that component of my films very seriously until I started work on my documentary *Black Gold: The Trail to Standing Rock.*

I found that I was wanted to be taken seriously as a filmmaker, so I had to up my game. I had to find my own collaborator who matched, individual, and musically, my own storytelling voice.

For *Letters to Daniel*, I wanted someone who was supremely talented, someone whose music was beautiful, layered, and conveyed deep emotion. In short, I needed a musical genius who had access to the kind of tools to make my film really pop. And, for the longest time, I avoided approaching composers because they cost a lot, at least any composer worth their salt.

I knew composers who would do it for an IMDB credit, where a short film was concerned. But *Letters* was a feature, and a feature film demanded pay.

During a time when I thought I had twenty grand to make the movie, I went to Indie Gathering in 2016, in search of my beautiful mind/musical genius.

While there, Ray introduced me to two composers, a nice young woman who was an honorable mention finisher, and Valyo Gennoff, who had placed second.

Valyo is a soft-spoken, incredibly modest, magnificently talented, Bulgarian composer. He is also incredibly sweet, and supportive, of all his fellow artists.

When Ray introduced me to him, and I heard his music, I thought, *There's no way I can afford this guy.* He was primetime ready straight out of the box. I still had (and still do) a lot to learn. I couldn't imagine someone as talented as Valyo wanting to work with the likes of me.

Come the award ceremony, like usual, everyone was packed into the room, waiting for the festivities to begin. That year, I won eleven awards. When you walk to the front of the room that many times, people may not remember your name, but they do remember your face, and I soon learned that they tended to want to work with you.

I got home from Indie Gathering that year but did not immediately send emails to all the people whom I had met. I was too busy getting ready for AOF (Action On Film) to send them anything yet. I did, however, receive an email between the time I got home from TIG and when I took off for AOF.

It was from Valyo. He wrote that he wanted to work with me, and he thought we would make a great team.

That fall, I shot *Broken* and used Kylie Jude for what would, most likely, be his last time as a composer. When I began work on a documentary, which was a real departure for me, I found that I was looking to make my mark and set my work apart from other filmmakers.

While just about everything behind the scenes on *Black Gold* was a disaster, the resulting product, and my working relationship with Valyo was not.

My working relationship with Valyo, (and Maria, my voice over talent) were the bright shining lights of my work experience on that film.

When Valyo sent me the introduction music, I got chills because it was so good. He far exceeded my hopes, and my expectations. He raised the level of professionalism on that film all on his own. Our film was screened at several festivals solely because of his score.

The documentary was solid. And, when I went to Indie Gathering, and AOF, I was rewarded for my efforts. I received Best Female Filmmaker-Feature, Best Director Documentary, Best Editing Documentary, and Best Soundtrack nominations for it. We took home Best Editing Documentary, and Valyo won Runner-Up for Best Soundtrack.

After such a killer outing, I knew that I wanted to work with Valyo whenever I could. When I got home from Vegas in 2017, I contacted Valyo and promptly invited him to score *Letters to Daniel* whenever we had a finished project. He immediately agreed.

That winter, he composed an intro to *Letters to Daniel*. It was so hauntingly beautiful that I cried. To think, my movie about my life, and my struggles with bipolar disorder, was going to have such gorgeous music attached to it thrilled me to no end!

As the years passed, I would make several low to no budget documentaries. Valyo would score them. I also shot *The Weekend* during this time, a romantic drama about how human trafficking impacts a married couple after a missing wife returns to her everyday life and finds it impossible to cope with life, and is unable to function properly in her marriage.

With each outing, Valyo more than proved himself up to the task of imbuing my work with the kind of pathos only music could bring. When listening to Valyo's work, I got excited because I knew that I was working with someone who helped make me better as a filmmaker; he lifted me up and praised my work.

Valyo is the kind of guy who would give the shirt off his back. And, when I told him he had to enter AOF and Hollywood Dreamz because it would change his life, he did. They, like they always do, embraced him with open arms.

I always write press releases for my work. I would happily write them for him if he asked me to. He's elevated the quality of my work on so many occasions that it behooves me to say, if anyone out there is looking for an amazing composer, then he's your guy.

He was the first person I signed on for *Letters to Daniel*. Through so many setbacks, pushbacks, close calls, he stuck by me and said that he still wanted to do it.

I couldn't get the local scene to respond to my cast and crew calls. Yet here was a guy, all the way in Bulgaria, who was willing to go that extra mile for me.

This moved me deeply. When you fall down and scrape up your hands and knees, simple human kindness is all that you really want. Valyo has that, in spades.

When I would panic about my project, Valyo would always have such encouraging words to share with me. He basically echoed what Missy was saying.

He said, "You have sown the seeds for a great harvest. God wouldn't bring you this far to just see the project die. You have worked hard, you're going reap an abundance of great things."

I told him that I certainly hoped so.

Letters has been a long, winding, hard and, ultimately, very rewarding road. One percent of filmmakers make their dream projects. I've done that. But I'm not satisfied with that, I'm still striving to reach the next level.

Seeing that *Letters to Daniel* is, at this writing, in post-production, I'm seeing how the rest of the journey plays out.

I wonder what the world will bring to my doorstep. As it is, I have been blessed to write up storm after four months of no writing.

Listening to Valyo's music is inspiring. When Valyo signed on, I knew that I couldn't run and gun shoot this thing. I needed a proper DP, a skilled editor, solid sound people. The budget for those things would be spread over time but, ultimately, it would cost every red cent that was in both mine and Missy's pockets, along with about two grand from crowdfunding.

What we spent was a drop in the bucket compared to most people, but it was a lot of money for us. We went all in; we cashed in all our chips, in the hope that this project would A, help people, B, educate people, and C, help launch our careers to the next level.

With someone like Valyo Gennoff on your team, you're well on your way there because people like Valyo are talented, have a strong worth ethic, and give their best every time out. They don't rest on their laurels, and they certainly don't give you excuses as to why something is not possible. If you say, "Make it so," Valyo is the kind of individual who will do everything humanly possible to make it happen.

When you're working in film, especially in indie film, you need collaborators who view things like the way you do. Everyone on my team serviced the story first. Everyone was unselfish, and gave straight from the heart.

Finding people like that is rare, finding as many as I did was even rarer.

I like to hold up Valyo as the bright, shining example that he is because I am so lucky to have answered his email. I stopped thinking of myself as unworthy.

One nice thing (among many nice things) about AOF is that I had (before I went in 2016) resigned myself to just writing screenplays and entering them into contests. Before AOF (and *Letters to Daniel*) I didn't deem myself as worthy of anything beyond those honorable mentions as a filmmaker.

You do it enough times, then you want to better yourself. And how do you do that? By educating yourself. "How?" You might ask. The obvious answer is film school. But, if you can't go to film school, read books, study film, and pick up a camera and go. What's stopping you?

Another way to better yourself is to surround yourself with people who are experienced enough so that you can learn from them. Through the production of *Letters to Daniel*, I learned so much. I'm still learning a lot in post-production, too. With Valyo, I handed him the final cut, and set him loose to do what it is he does so well.

Valyo was the first talent to believe in me and Missy and *Letters to Daniel*. We couldn't wait to hear what he had in store for the film.

6

MISSY GOODMAN: CO-WRITER, CO-CONSPIRATOR, CAREGIVER & SUPERHERO

I know I previously said that Valyo was the first one on board but, really, for *Letters to Daniel* to even be a thing means that I had to have lived through fire to be able to share what it was like in the there. The only reason I did so was because of Missy Goodman.

One cannot overstate what role Missy has played in my recovery. When a person is going through the unique hell that is bipolar disorder, it puts everyone in its direct path at risk. The impulsive, irrational behavior that comes along with the disease puts everyone through their paces.

While I felt like dying, Missy was forced to contend with a very sick individual. Not that I was evil. Not a lunatic, or "crazy," just sick. The world would be a much better place if people just showed one another simple human kindness.

Initially, Missy struggled with it as much as I did. Where had her bright and cheery friend gone? Who was this broken creature who had taken her place?

Caregiver.

I've often searched for the proper word for what Missy's role in my life has been, and it has changed over the years.

Initially, we worked together at B. Dalton Bookseller's, where both of us gained our love of reading, and that was when we began to write stories, and cast them. Every day, I was scheduled to work with her, I made sure that she had something new of mine to read. She would then share her stories orally. In the beginning, however, she would never let me read her stuff.

After a whole year of this, she approached me to write a romance novel with her.

I very arrogantly said, "Yeah, let's do it for the money." I was twenty-one years old. Little did I know that, eventually, I would cut my storytelling teeth in sub-genre romance, as it were, and we got started.

That first unpublished novel had an endless outline, and the only things salvageable were the memorable heroines, Ariel and Adriana Stuart. They would stay with us over the years, being written into many different incarnations. Sometimes, we would lie around and verbally add layers to it.

The second incarnation of it would be a feature length script. Needless to say, both of those items were long gone.

Some of the first signs that something wasn't right included insomnia, the inability to be alone, and sudden emotional outbursts at odd times.

But we were so busy writing that we didn't see the oncoming freight train.

It was amazing what Missy and I had managed to accomplish in the wake of such devastation and, believe me, bipolar disorder is a devastating disease. It sneaks in and, if you're not aware of your triggers, or situations that put you at risk, then it will shatter your life into a million little pieces and send those around you through the emotional wringer, again and again and again.

Having had our friendship tested by the fires of mental illness, poverty, and hunger, there was not much out there that Missy and I couldn't handle together. So, when I went to Missy about the idea of writing about our struggles with my disease, she was understandably hesitant at first. Who willingly airs their most vulnerable moments for public digestion, and discussion?

No one wants to come off as the self-indulgent, famous for being famous, Kardashians, especially when talking about a subject as serious as mental illness. When you choose to share your story, it should be one of consequence, not where you quibbling and putting your dysfunctional lives on display just for fame and fortune, especially when you already have both.

There needs to be a healing component to your story, or else you're just like any other glory hog who wants nothing more than a reality television show for their family.

I want *Letters to Daniel* to play more like *A Beautiful Mind* and less like the Duggars. From what I can tell, however, it already does.

It took a while for Missy to come around and see things my way, a couple of weeks. During which time, a rough draft of the screenplay was burning out of control inside of me. In retrospect, Missy said she just needed time to get her head around it because she knew that, for some reason, I needed to tell my story, and that I was pretty much going to do it, anyway.

Co-Conspirator.

When I told Missy that I wanted produce and direct the

screenplay, she resisted. She said that did not enjoy that part and would be happy just to be the writer.

At first, I had shopped it around to some of the indie film-makers whom we had met at Indie Gathering. Some said that it would take two solid weeks to make the movie the way that it needed to be made. Others said that it would cost too much money. I even had one idiot say, "You need 75K to make this happen, why don't you submit it to Amazon?" He was full of shit, and he let us down when it came to filming our micro short.

Ultimately, it was just all white noise to me. To those individuals, they were giving me legit reasons why they couldn't possibly do it. To me, they were just excuses from people who just weren't interested in helping me produce my script. Not all of those people were bad, thought. Some were writer/directors who only wanted to make their own films. Ultimately, however, all those people were useless to me.

Which brought me back to Missy. This time, when I asked her to produce, she said, "Yes." And, through all the setbacks from the summer of 2015, up until when we finally filmed the beast of a thing during the summer of 2019, she stuck by my side.

Through the disaster of the film falling apart in 2015, to my nearly losing my shit with corrupt, toxic, and abusive management in 2016, and the false promise of 20K to make my dream project in 2017, Missy never wavered in her support, even if she did doubt my sanity during some instances.

Co-Writer.

Before we were friends, we were co-writers. What we started out with were weekly meetings, where we shared and edited our solo projects with each other. Shortly after, we began meeting every night to co-write. I said that the only rule we had to abide by was to watch *The X-Files* before we began any work.

Missy wasn't sure she liked that idea. The only episode she had ever watched was "To Jose Chung From Outer Space." Charles Nelson Riley was the guest star, and it was a comical look at the absurdity that *The X-Files* really was.

Fortunately, it was a monster of the week episode, and Missy said that she loved it (maybe not as much as me) and, thus, our beautiful partnership was born.

On Mother's Day 1999, we traveled to Charles Town, WV to hand our first co-written script to Maurice Benard (Sonny Corinthos, *General Hospital*, *The Ghost and the Whale*). It was a crazy experience.

At the time, I had begun to suspect that, maybe, I might have bipolar disorder, but I didn't want to self-diagnose, and I was too afraid to go and have myself checked out. It had been my experience that, although stigma exists for all mental illnesses, it's still more acceptable to call yourself depressed, or to say that you have PTSD, than it is to say you have anxiety. When you say that you have bipolar disorder, (thanks to the way certain tragedies are sensationalized by news media, and how the first thing out of their mouths is he had bipolar disorder) it's seen as an unfixable, unpleasant thing about you. In the beginning, when I said that I had bipolar disorder, people would give you "the look." The one that says, *"Oh, my God, you're a crazy person."*

Even when it was terrible, and I was crying all night and I couldn't function, Missy may have been pushed to the brink, and didn't understand all the time, but she always found a way to show me compassion. And, when I was at my sickest, she never once ran from the fight that the disease put up.

Superhero.

Caregivers are the unsung heroes in the battle against the stigma, the mental illness, itself, and the daily care of those of us who are diagnosed with it.

They often have battles of their own related specifically to caregiving. What Missy does is simply amazing: she goes to school, she owns a publishing house, she does Poshmark, and she helps me pursue my dreams while steadying me so that I can truly soar.

Missy is under no obligation to help me at all. We're not related. We're not married. She stood by me for a lot of reasons. First of all, she told me that her father always said, "Goodmans don't run."

To which she playfully added, "Even when they should, sometimes." She said that I always getting treatment. And, maybe, we were each a little bit co-dependent.

In the end, we made it through to other side in part because, when we moved to Texas (that's right, not California, smooth move on our part) to make a movie, we had absolutely no idea what we were headed into.

If we had any idea about the storm that would brew, I doubt we would have taken the journey that we did. And, if we hadn't, *Letters to Daniel* wouldn't be a thing, and we wouldn't be standing we are right now, with a finished film, and our careers about to explode.

7

CLINT GAIGE: AOFER, FRIEND, MENTOR, EDITOR

𝒶 OF really is the gift that keeps on giving. I've been fortunate to have people who have supported me. But I really didn't find success as a writer until I was thirty-five, in film, until I was thirty-nine, and they were all from the independent film festival scene. Indie Gathering gave me some team players, and they were great. With Valyo standing out as a composer, and Brandon Bell being the dream actor.

As a member of AOF's Class of 2016, I met Clint twice in passing during that same year. AOF was in Monrovia, CA. I once saw him walking through the corridor of the Krikorian movie theater. He was super nice, and effusive.

He then shouted over to me, "I'm sorry I didn't get to your movie, but I believe in what you're doing; keep on doing it."

I met him again after the awards ceremony, when he had won for Best Action Sequence in a Feature. I had won for Best Social Commentary with my *Letters to Daniel: Breakdown to Bestseller* documentary. We friended each other on Facebook and, then, we began a live friendship, and which blossomed into him giving me feedback. And all that had finally led to a working relationship.

Somewhere during that time, I asked him to be the editor for *Letters to Daniel*, and he agreed.

For a while, it seemed like my film would never get made. I knew that Clint had said yes but Clint, like Mark, worked in the industry, so he was a professional. He was in demand, and he was in demand for a reason. He had twenty-two years' experience, and it showed in his directorial work.

In 2017, at AOF, I had more of a chance to sit down and talk with him. There was a conversation at one of the bars in the Palms near the Brendan Theaters. It was late, and Rebekah and I were coming from a screening.

We ran into Clint and one of his actors, Konstantine James, (I think that is his name) and we talked about *Fat Guy with a Shotgun* (Clint's film) and the state of *Letters to Daniel*, my microfilm, my proof of concept trailer, and my short, *Broken and Black Gold: The Trail to Standing Rock*.

I would learn that Clint was starting up his own film festival, the Enginuity Film Festival, and that he was judging the Clifton Film Celebration. In a way that only Clint can, he managed to talk me into entering both festivals. There was no favoritism shown, like at AOF; Clint's festival, and CFC, are festivals with integrity.

I would get honest feedback about where my film shined, and where it needed work. Clint has become something of a mentor to me. In 2017, I was nominated at the Clifton Film Celebration for Best Feature Documentary and the Do the Thing Award. I wouldn't win either, but I was thrilled just to be nominated.

At Enginuity, I would receive praise for the way that I handled the subject matter, the voice talent, and the score. I wouldn't be selected, or nominated, but the feedback by a PBS judge was just as valuable, if not more so than had I got selected, or nominated.

When picking a topic for my next documentary, I looked at bipolar disorder, how it affects everyone in the family, and how it is genetic. I interviewed my mom and dad. I prepared the interview questions, and my cousin, Rebekah, interviewed me. Then, I interviewed her and my Aunt Jan, who just so happens to be her grandmother.

I took some b-roll, still photography, and wrote as tight a script for a documentary that I could. I hired Maria Christian to do the narration.

When I sent it to Clint for some feedback, he said, "You know, this needs a good color grade."

I said, "Okay," and hired him to do it for me.

When I got my film back, I was flabbergasted at the difference from his suggestion. The name of the documentary was *All in the Family*, and it did extremely well on the festival circuit.

I was at a loss in some ways. I didn't have much money to speak of and, when it would come time for *Letters to Daniel*, I would find lots of willing participants, except for where sound was concerned.

I wanted the best. But the best cost $2,800 dollars, plus shelter, gas, and food. Unless he let me pay him in installments, I wouldn't be able to do it, and it just doesn't work like that in the film industry.

Fortunately, I would find the people to run boom, but I still wish I could have afforded a brilliant sound guy. I think every indie filmmaker wishes they had a brilliant sound guy. Usually, however, they don't, but that's for another chapter.

During the past three years, I feel like Clint had taken me

under his wing and taught me a lot about how a filmmaker/editor relationship works. There's a give and take and, when I started on *Letters to Daniel*, I would soon discover was that Clint is always working to better himself as a filmmaker. During the filming of *Letters to Daniel*, he told me that he was taking a master colorist class. Then, he showed me an example of his work.

I was freaking excited. The quality, and level of professionalism, in the before and after frames was incredible. I was thrilled beyond words. I knew that my film was going to be beautiful.

What followed were conversations between Clint and Mark and myself, discussing the state of mine and Missy's film.

The first thing to be addressed was sound. It was recorded at an extremely low level. Like at -36, as opposed to the normal -6. It left my editor stymied, and Mark and Clint openly talked about ADR.

Mark had been pushing for it. I was getting comfortable with idea of scheduling thirty-five people to go to Arkansas when Mark announced I would also have to do Foley, that is, add in all the sounds: footsteps, doors closing, etc. Chances were that I was leaving it in the hands of my brilliant composer to clean up the sound. Remember, Hal had atrocious sound, and he performed a minor miracle with it.

I was supposed to see a cut of the film that night, and I was anxious and excited.

Letters to Daniel had been a labor of love, dating back to May 7, 2013. Having launched the *Letters* blog on that date, some would say the journey began then. But I honestly think that it really dates back as far as shortly before Missy and I left for San Antonio, TX when I was becoming symptomatic, and didn't know it.

Missy always said that, if she had it to do over again, she wouldn't have moved. She also said that she would have stayed in Kentucky, forced a co-worker out of a position the Missy had earned, and gotten a place to live, and found me the help that I needed.

I don't regret our time in Texas. It made us into who we are today. I don't believe that things happen for reason. We live in a much too random of a world for that to be true. I believe that every decision you make in your life brings you to where you are today.

Because I saw *Casino Royale*, I was inspired to cast Daniel Craig (physically) as the hero in *Another Way to Die*. Everything grew from that creative seed. When Missy's father was in the hospital, slowly declining in health, I chose to submit my script to the Ozarks Film Festival, and my *Another Way to Die* manuscript to Lyrical Press.

Those were my first projects featuring Daniel Craig-inspired heroes. While the script died, the book would find a home with MuseItUp Publishing.

Several more books would follow. Twenty-four titles have been published so far, with two coming out this fall and four others completed and one contracted for.

From 2013 on, we've completed thirty-two scripts, all of which have won awards, which led me to believe the decision to go all in at AOF in 2016 was the most important career decision that I could have made. They gave me a foundation to stand on when there were others taking advantage of me. They gave me the courage to keep striving until, finally, I had the whole team that I wanted and said, "Fuck the naysayers, I'm going to do this."

Men at other festivals said that, "As long as you insist on directing your film, then you will never get it made." Del and

Theresa were at the other end of the spectrum, saying, "Fuck those people. You've got the talent, go for it."

To be honest, I survived childhood sex abuse, and I do battle with bipolar disorder on a daily basis. People telling me that I can't do things is just some bullshit I've been told all my life. I may get distracted sometimes but, eventually, I'm able to refocus and just get what I need to done.

Clint Gaige is a genius, though he says he's only smart enough to know that he needs to learn more. That's the mark of a humble, talented, man.

In the wake of the #Me Too Movement, I considered having an all-female crew. But I realized that I had been building an Indie Gathering/AOF crew and, if that meant having a few more guys, then I was good with that.

I always put the film first.

As the production ended, it was imperative for me to get the footage to Clint. We were on a tight schedule. But, when I realized that it wouldn't be ready in time, or be at its best, I took my finger off the proverbial trigger.

The following morning seemed to be the delivery time for the first cut of the movie. Clint lives out in the boonies, so that makes using the Internet challenging, especially for large projects, like films over fifty minutes that you want to email your client.

Sometimes, I think I've got crap Internet service. Then, I work with Clint, and I'm reminded that some have it better, and others have it worse. And even though Clint has it worse, he's not much on complaining about it, which makes him strong.

I finally spent the largest chunk of time with Clint at the Hollywood Dreamz Award Show and Dinner. The food was delish, and the entertainment killer. The jazz legend, Jimmy Mulidore, as well as the conversation, was sparkling.

I sat with the three men whom I knew would ultimately determine my film's fate. Clint Gaige, a filmmaker who got his start in the industry editing a talk show for a local television channel, Mark Maness, a cinematographer who has been plying his trade since 1986, and Valyo Gennoff, a musical savant who travelled twenty-two hours just to attend the debut of the film which he scored for me.

Hard to believe it took another year and a half, but we finally made *Letters to Daniel*, and it was unlike anything I'd ever experienced!

8

MARK MANESS: SOUTHERNER, CINEMATOGRAPHER/GENIUS

*A*ction On Film, Class of 2016, take 2. I met Mark Maness as I was heading to watch a film, and Mark was headed to one of the many inspirational seminars that AOF is known for. Brilliant writers, filmmakers, actors, producers; you name them, they have them.

We stopped, and I asked what movie he was there with. If I recall, it was *Birthrite*; I'd have to ask Mark just to be completely sure.

He asked me the same thing.

Then, because of his distinctive accent I asked him where he was from.

"Arkansas," he replied.

I told him that I was from the South, too.

"Really, where are *you* from?" he asked, his curiosity piqued.

"Kentucky," I replied.

"That ain't the South," he said.

"You'd better not tell anyone from Kentucky that."

We both laughed, and our friendship took off from there.

We talked for a few more minutes and then parted company. We met up again when we both attended Del Weston's Get It Done: From Script to Screen seminar. We took notes and talked about how amazing the festival was.

I finally told him what my film was about, and that it was nominated, but I also said that I didn't expect to win at such a large festival, and I was just grateful to be invited to the party.

Mark and I were both at the Writers Awards Dinner, where he won for *It Know* (a brilliant psychological thriller) script, and now film. I won for Best New Writer at AOF, and I got emotional. To be recognized for my work among the extremely talented screenwriters who were in the room, and at such a big event, was simply overwhelming.

I managed to hold myself together for the speech but, when I sat down, I received a beautiful text message from another attendee, and the floodgates opened. My dear friends, James and Andrew, were there when that happened. Me and Missy were fighting to break through to the next level. To know that a West Coast festival saw something special in us was a heady feeling.

Then, there was the black tie AOF Awards Show and Dinner held at the Westin Hotel Ballroom in Pasadena, CA. I was seriously out of my element. In pants and a blouse and tennis shoes, I was seriously underdressed for the affair.

Del personally seated us, (Bob and Jackie Messinger and Rich McKee) and everyone else, at the table. (Everyone who was nominated at the table would be winners by the end of the night.)

Right as they got to my category, Best Social Commentary, Rich leaned over and said, "Everyone else has won. You're going to win."

I told him to be quiet. I doubted that I would get anything. I thought that, if I got anything, that it would be a runner up. So, when someone else's name was announced as the winner, I would just smile and think, *Oh, well, it was nice to be nominated.*

Then, Del said, "*Letters to Daniel.*"

Oh, shit; now I have to go up there and actually say something, I thought.

Anabelle Munro remembers an eloquent speech. I just remember giving Del a hug, and my speech going by in a blur. There were a lot of people in that room. And, truth be told, I had never spoken in front of such a large crowd.

Mark would win that night, too. I sought him out after the ceremony, and we snapped a photo together then said our good-byes. Shortly after I got home, I messaged Mark on FB and asked him if he would DP the narrative version of *Letters to Daniel,* and he accepted.

It would be three more years before we would move on *Letters to Daniel,* but Mark was a great mentor. He would always answer my questions, give me advice about how to make my movies come alive, and notes about how to make them more cinematically appealing while adhering to my original vision.

Letters to Daniel, the screenplay, was doing well on the circuit. There were only two places where it hadn't been officially selected, the Austin Film Festival and ARFF, and the Austin Revolution Film Festival.

I believed in the script. It was the single most emotionally powerful, and personal, thing I had ever written with Missy. We laid our souls bare, and made ourselves completely vulnerable. The festivals weren't wrong for not choosing us. Contests are so subjective, so you really don't know, from festival to festival, what they'll like. I'd gotten selected at ARFF for the past two years with other scripts, and a proof of concept trailer. They're an amazing festival; their purpose is to elevate the indie film-maker and create a community where *filmmakers* help one another make films against the grain.

I haven't had the chance to attend ARFF, but I hope to next year. Should the finances hold out, and *Letters to Daniel* get accepted there.

ARFF is Mark, and his beautiful wife, Janet's, favorite festi-val. I can't wait to go to ARFF, but AOF aligns more with my ambitions, to break through to the mainstream. I've yet to see a festival which is matched with taking damaged artists, restoring their confidence while showering them with love, and setting them up to believe whatever path they strike out on is legitimate.

While AOF can't guarantee mainstream success, they can give you the proper tools you'll need to make the effort to get there.

Love and human kindness is in great supply at both AOF, and ARFF. But it was AOF which got behind me with mentor-ship, and helped in bettering myself as a screenwriter, and film-maker. AOF enabled me to draw the kind of talent Mark Maness is (he's a freaking genius) to *Letters to Daniel*.

I would attend AOF in 2017, when it moved to the Palms in Las Vegas, so would Mark and Janet. We would spend a lot of time together and take many business meals. Me, Thomas Moore, Rebekah, Mark, Janet, Ana Jobrail, and Valyo Gennoff spent a lot of time together. We all determined that we were combined to make the perfect team.

Mark and Janet were a blast to hang out with. When I finally asked Mark to be DP, he agreed.

In 2018, I endeavored to make it to his place, but his hectic schedule, (He would catch hell from his boss for taking a week's vacation before an annual trade show to do *Letters*.) and my tight budget for film, made that an impossibility.

No problem. I searched for a producer, but I never really found one. I did find someone who raised money, and he also promoted. That guy likes to take credit for work he had no part in, but that's Mark for you.

As AOF 2018 rolled around, he was unable to make the festival. I put on my big girl panties and made it happen. Although, truthfully, the bipolar disorder was kicking me hard. For the record, Missy is the Producer with a capital "P." I'm the director, and she and I are co-writers on the script.

I made AOF this year by the skin of my teeth. Mark came down to Kentucky and, once he arrived at the motel, he said that it looked sketchy. He was afraid to leave his film truck parked there, and I couldn't really blame him. He said, "Amy, if it wasn't for you, I would have turned around and gone straight back to Arkansas."

Intown Suites. 7121 Preston Hwy, in Louisville, KY. Bugs on the pillow. Mold in the shower. Paper thin towels that you have to pay four dollars to have cleaned. After one roll of toilet paper, you had to replace it on your own.

They say that's indie film.

I'm fortunate that my small, yet dedicated, crew did not abandon me before the day, and our call to action.

To say Mark has a low bullshit threshold is something of an understatement; he's all about getting the work done. Thank God that we were the perfect match for those six days. I made everyone bust their asses and, fortunately, they didn't revolt.

There were several instances where they could have. On the last day, Missy nearly walked off the set. I had pushed her to her breaking point and embarrassed her. But, in all reality, on the last day working hard in ninety-one degree heat and high humidity, I was surprised that I could control my temper and anxiety at all.

Maybe, on some level, I knew what awaited me if I did push people too hard.

As it was, Mark and my crew worked miracles, and I now have a beautiful film as a result. And my leads, Megan Jones, and Virginia, rose to the occasion and performed better than I could have imagined.

Mark is the epitome of what a southern gentleman is in the grandest sense of the word. He treats woman like ladies, and as equals. Never once did I feel like he was directing my film. I felt like Mark was busting his rear-end to give me the best movie possible, and the result was gorgeous.

Do I wish this genius would slow his roll a little in post? Yes, but I know that he's not creating a mutiny on my film; he truly is working to give me the best of his talents, and I can only be grateful for that.

Mark's expertise in filmmaking far exceeds cinematography, it stretches into sound design, as he is also a guitar and bass player.

Mark could rock 'n' roll with the best of them. We were able to shoot the movie at such a breakneck pace because of Mark's extensive education, and experience. Like he once posted, *You don't pay for the fact I can accomplish what you want in thirty minutes, you pay me for how long it took me to learn how to do it in thirty minutes.*

At the time, Mark was engineering his breakthrough with the amazing *It Knows*, which stars Lauren Lasseigne, Carmen Patterson, and Dan Michael. Dan gives a chilling portrayal of an abusive father with murderous impulses. Carmen gives a riveting portrayal of a woman tortured by her past, and mental illness. And Lauren Lasseigne simply commands the screen anytime that she's on it. Mark's masterful direction of this film is what won me over, for good, when it came to deciding who would be my director of photography. Mark is a genius. And, because of his generosity, and talent, my dream came true; that cannot be said enough.

9

FINDING THE MONEY

I've been singing AOF's praises. Now, it's time to talk about Indie Gathering's influence on me as a film-maker, and a screenwriter. It seems, at every festival, that there are tiers of talent. Indie Gathering is no different. But, like AOF, they do their own thing, and what Indie Gathering is truly known for is networking.

It took four years of attending with various (forty-five) projects until we went to William John's film which, for the life of me I couldn't remember the name of, with hopes of him producing *Letters to Daniel*.

We sat through the film. Like Mark's, it wasn't really my cup of tea, but it was very well-done. I got a hold of him afterwards and said that I'd like to buy him a drink and talk to him about *Letters to Daniel*.

He had Peter John Ross come along, and we all went to the lounge and got a round of drinks, except for Ross, he had French fries.

It quickly became clear that William had little interest in

producing a feature. He was getting ready to dive, head first, into fatherhood again, (the baby is adorable) and his free time was at a premium. He volunteered Ross for the job.

Ross begged off, but he also said that there was a producer in Cincinnati whom he thought might be a good fit. His name was Aaron Allen.

We enjoyed the drink and fries and went our separate ways. Last year at Indie Gathering, I had less than a stellar time, but let me reiterate that it had nothing to do with the hosts of the festival, or the festival itself.

My bipolar disorder was flaring, and I was symptomatic. I wasn't feeling the love, (we won eleven awards there last year) but, when you're symptomatic, big crowds, sleep deprivation, and the way your bipolar brain works can really send you into a downward spiral of obsessive thoughts and paranoia. Or even mixed mania, where you loathe yourself, and your mind won't slow down.

Fortunately, Missy was with me, caring for me. Thanks to her, I relented and let Ray sit me down with Ricardo Raymundo. I friended Aaron on FB, and he immediately asked to see the script.

Within days of our return from Indie Gathering, he said that he would like to produce the film. While he wouldn't function as a producer with a capital "P," he would work as a great promoter of the *Letters to Daniel* brand, and would help us to raise more money for our film than we ever had before.

Aaron has a good heart in most respects, and he was great at generating fundraisers, but he stepped on the toes of more than one of my crew members in the process. That forced me to have to be the bad guy with him and to smooth over any ruffled feathers.

When we were securing locations, he said that he had an

apartment which we could use. Then, when we got closer to the actual filming date, that fell through, and he wanted me to house my cast and crew in a warehouse.

What I did house them in was far from ideal, but was a warehouse some stranger fancied he could turn into a movie studio overnight any better? It was at that point when I wrested control of the *Letters to Daniel* machine back and found two places which would serve as good locations.

Aaron did a magnificent job of drawing people to donate to the film. Two grand was more than anything we'd raised before. But, even though there were actresses, and money, coming from his community, a majority would come from the writing and filmmaking connections that Missy and I had made over the years. Friends, family, even my church gave to the cause that was *Letters to Daniel*.

What started as a fan letter then turned into a blog and had blossomed into way more than I could ever imagine.

Letters to Daniel had been a six-year journey. There was the festival tour and distribution leg of the journey. And this memoir and touring with it.

Sometimes, I wondered if *Letters to Daniel* would be over. I'm so in creative love with what we had filmed over the course of six days, and we really couldn't have done it without the two grand.

Aaron was a fundraising beast. Everyone was a beast.

Aaron always checked in and shared the photos and dug the poster. The truth is that it took everyone to make our little miracle of a movie, and to make it amazing all around.

But, it started with the first yes, and Aaron said, "Yes."

Previously, I had attended ICFF. Now, ICFF had born *Letters to Daniel* a lot of opportunities, such as its first nomination. And it was because of ICFF that I made a calculated decision to remove all swear words from the script. I decided the story stood strong on its own, in spite of the subtractions.

As it was, two curse words survived, and in the same scene. Both were spoken by Missy, which is ironic because I'm the one with a bit of a potty mouth. But we both agree that our favorite curse word is any variation of the word fuck.

Nothing is quite as powerful as that word for getting a point across, and the first draft of the script was peppered liberally with it. If I was going to enter it into ICFF, those f-bombs, along with a lot of other words, had to go.

It turned out to be the smartest decision that I made regarding the script. It garnered a lot of nominations and official selections and a couple of wins. And it caught the eye of ParablesTV/Upliftv executive, Isaac Hernandez.

In March of 2018, I contacted Isaac online, through Facebook, and I asked him if I could pick his brain.

He said, "Yes" then gave me his number, and we set up a time to talk.

During that time, I pitched to him both *The Guardian* and *Letters to Daniel*. He told me to send him the scripts, and we made a plan to meet up and talk in Nashville.

Now, I had to figure out how to get to Nashville. He was attending NRB. I'll be frank, I didn't see the point of attending that convention. But, when he walked up he gave me a big hug, he was full of positive energy.

His words were very simple, and to the point. He said, "Amy, I've read about two-thirds of *Letters to Daniel*. All I can say is that you're unstoppable, and your friend is amazing. Here's what I'm going to do for you. I'm going to put you on ParablesTV/Upliftv. We'll set up a revenue share. There are several other faith-based networks I have relationships with, I'll use them to get your film on those platforms."

I was gobsmacked. I still wanted theatrical and DVD. But I was walking out of there with at least one avenue of distribution in my hip pocket. I rode a Greyhound to both there and back from Louisville. My day started at seven in the morning, and ended at close to midnight.

I ended that day on such a high.

I would go into the ICFF feeling confident. When I pitched *Letters to Daniel* to would-be producers there, they spoke another language. They spoke in terms of "ministry" not "art." I had a studio head tell me that she'd heard of *Letters to Daniel*. I spoke with her for a good forty-five minutes.

I pitched *Letters to Daniel* to her, and she bought the book. Other producers would initially nibble but would ultimately tell me their versions of, "No." Some were condescending, saying, "As long as you insist on directing it, it will never get made." Others were more dismissive of me outright, saying, "I always tell screenwriters not to pass up an opportunity when it presents itself. But, if the Lord is calling you to direct this movie, then, by all means, direct it."

What the hell was that supposed to mean?

If God deemed it so? How arrogant was he (the producer) to think God that ordained him Lord, God of film, and I was what, God's afterthought?

Screw him, and everyone else there who stigmatized me, dismissed me, or said, "Pray it away." You can't pray mental illness away. Prayer and meditation are tools in the tool belt during times of crisis and can be used to implement, with medication, therapy, and the support of friends and family true healing.

Letters to Daniel was the final step in achieving and maintaining a life of rolling hills, instead of crazy, out of control rollercoaster rides. Prayer isn't the silver bullet answer to mental illness.

Even though I was stigmatized, I knew that I was meant to be there. I just needed to reach one person in the audience and inspire them to get help.

Isaac had become a champion. When Aaron set-up the GoFundMe, Isaac was one of the first ones to donate. It's an incredible feeling to have an executive get behind you and encourage you to achieve your dreams.

In the end, the film had financially put the screws to both Missy and me. But, when you believe in yourself and have supporters at your back, then there is no limit to what you can do.

Missy has famously said, "Amy, I believe we can do anything that you put your mind to."

"Certain avenues of distribution has intimated they're open to and Emmy campaign for *Letters to Daniel*, and certain principal subjects involved."

"That would be fabulous. Is there a chance we could get lost in the major television network shuffle? Maybe. But I've found that, when you put your desires out into the universe and put action behind it, amazing things can happen."

"It looks like I will have a couple of more shows that ParablesTV/Upliftv will want, *Recovery Unplugged* and *The Guardian*. One's a mental health/creative arts talk show, and the other one is faith-based and takes aim at stigma in the Christian faith. I'm a Christian, but I have experienced stigma in the faith. *Letters to Daniel* seeks to address stigma everywhere."

Finding the money was a Godsend. Getting the movie made was a miracle, one which I am blessed to have experienced.

DOUG KAUFMAN: SCRIPT SUPERVISOR, PRE-PRODUCTION GOD

*D*oug Kaufman, aka. Dylan Francis Calvi, is a unique individual. He is something of a mad scientist. He's a veritable bull in a china shop and, if you run afoul of his personality, then you might find yourself running into a buzz saw.

But Doug is an effusive, emotional, and devoted guy. When working on a project, he puts 110 percent into it and answers every call to work. During pre-production, he was a dream to work with. I asked him to come on board as script supervisor; I honestly had no idea what to expect.

I'd met Doug at the 2016 Indie Gathering, and he'd been warm and acted as if we'd known each other forever. Then, we struck up a friendship online and would trade scripts and give each other feedback.

It was clear that he was an amazing writer and looking to make a move into directing and acting. He eventually signed a deal with Legacyverse. I don't know where that stands now. He is ninety-percent of the way through getting his feature directorial debut, *Tell Your Children*, (a tongue-in-cheek remake of

Reefer Madness) and has written several scripts which have done well at Horror Hotel and Indie Gathering.

Horror Hotel is his regular haunt, and he sometimes lands at Indie Gathering. And, in 2016, when I was feeling a bit wounded, I had encountered toxic shady people, and I wanted the world to know that I was not defeated.

Doug was just so sweet. Never in a million years did I think that I would connect with him and have him join me on the pre-production of *Letters to Daniel*.

When I asked him to come aboard the *Letters to Daniel* train, I didn't know what to expect. Doug has that wild man mentality, and we certainly don't see eye to eye on some subjects, but Doug was an answer to my prayers.

As soon as he said yes, he went and studied up on what a script supervisor's duties were. Shortly, he learned what to do, my production was streamlined, and organized, within an inch of its life.

I had the cast list, the script broken down, a streamlined shot list, and a shot-marked script. I was more prepared than I had ever been for any other film. If I needed anything, Doug was there to provide it.

Letters to Daniel was my all in gamble, and Doug seemed to inherently know that, and anticipated any, and all, pre-production needs.

The more I prepared, the more I knew that the on-set production was going to be murder. We were going to film a feature in eight days, which was insane to contemplate, but there was the reality.

Missy could only get so many days off. We had use of certain locations for a finite amount of time, and we only had so much money. A lot was riding on this production.

As the date of production neared, I grew increasingly

stressed out. My mood became more expansive. I became more irritable, and unstable. For four months, I didn't write a word. Everything was dedicated to the production of *Letters to Daniel*. If the risk did not pay off, it would have been especially painful.

This was my life story. I was pushing myself to the brink of my abilities, and my sanity, to make my swing for the fences. If it didn't pay off, I would have been devastated on several levels.

It was imperative that I have a team who knew this and was willing to go on the ride with me.

As of 2014, I often say that I'm the queen of making chicken salad out of chicken shit. And my films at Indie Gathering were perennial honorable mentions, but that didn't seem to matter to Doug. He read the script for *Letters to Daniel* and was all in.

Meanwhile, Missy bore the brunt of my instability. Initially, she didn't want to tell this story. In fact, I still don't know if she was thrilled about it. Putting your life experiences out there for people to judge, and comment on, is admittedly rough.

During the course of filming, it became clear to me that our little film had the potential to do amazing things.

On set, Doug was a devoted, and dedicated, member of the crew, even if he did drive me crazy with some of the things that he did. He provided me with his station wagon, Buck, the Big Brown Beast, for certain shots in the movie. But he refused to allow the voice over to be read, and didn't back up the footage, even after he was repeatedly told to do so.

Doug is a mad genius. His personality can rankle others on the set.

But, here's the thing, he didn't complain about the motel. He cooked, every night, at the end of thirteen-hour shooting days and happily spent every night transferring the footage so that I could email it to Clint.

So, even though I became very irritated with him at times, he's still a good friend, and I'm really happy for him. Thanks to his own work and, now, his performance of *Letters to Daniel*, he's parlayed that into paid work.

I'm hoping to parlay *Letters to Daniel* into paid work. Strong distribution deals, and maybe funding for a pilot talk show. All very ambitious, I know, but I think it's all very doable. And it all stems from good, clean, organizational skills on Doug's part.

During preparation time, I would video chat him regularly. I would ramble on and talk about nothing but *Letters to Daniel*.

During the buildup to June 2019, we had actually tried to produce the film in 2015. I wanted so much for the Louisville film community to embrace us. But the sad fact is that they have not. I have tried, over the years, to reach out to them. I even had three Louisville-based actors on set.

Then, about a week after filming, a local director, who shall remain nameless, emerged from that underbelly and tried to take me down a peg.

He informed me that, while I had "done a good job," I wasn't in the same class as the others in the area who regularly sacrificed their marriages, and mortgages, to do what they do. I was only able to pull it off because of charity, and taxpayers, and I owed them a collective, "Thank you." He then went on to say he owned his shit because he put it on credit, (that would mean the bank owned it, not him) and that he, not I, owned *Letters to Daniel*.

To say that I was blindsided would be an understatement. It was late. To be honest, I didn't know him all that well. I had met him at a local convention where I watched his film. It was poorly written, poorly directed, and poorly acted. His work is shit.

But it still stung. But, after I told my supporters of this incident, they reminded me that I had just achieved something only one percent of filmmakers ever do. Write, direct, and produce their passion project. And it was a feature film which, most likely, would have distribution and be a festival hit. What the hell had he accomplished?

What helped a lot was when the 2019 AOF Film and Video Nominations came out. I was to receive the Founder's Award for my body of work.

This director probably had a serious case of sour grapes. In retrospect, I realized that it must be miserable to live that way, to always be bitter in the face of someone else's success. How terrible to believe that one is superior to another and harbor such ill will. That kind of stuff rots you from the inside out.

Doug is not like that. On set one night, he sacrificed sleep just the get the files transferred to the extended hard drive so that I could get the first half of the footage mailed off to Clint. Then, he proceeded to collapse.

When we arrived at Mysti Parker's home, we found him lying down in the grass, with his arm over his eyes. It was day four, and we would be a man down when I asked Mysti if there was a place for him to lie down in the house.

He had been running on zero hours of sleep. Missy would be the set mom. When he broke down crying, she comforted him. Being the director, and somewhat hanging by my fingernails, myself, I was unable to give any TLC.

I was totally focused on filming my movie. Get the takes. Get the performances. By the end of the day, Doug was back up on his feet, but not really functioning. He and Caitlyn Druck (slate/make-up) fell off the face of the filmmaking earth altogether.

The nice thing is that we got some incredible footage of

Megan, Ginny, and Brandon. After our final shot of the day, I was spent, my feet were aching, so I wanted to chop them off. My brain was fried. I was spent. So I told Missy, "Be the director." I trusted her.

Megan and Michael would deliver on the funniest moment in the film. In a serious movie about a serious topic, there were several little moments of levity which helped make the movie flow and not feel like a grind.

Doug recovered by the next day, and it was awesome. By him having to step away for a day, it enabled Abigail (our 1 AD) to team up with Missy and supervise the script, and she would read the voice over to get proper timing. By the time Doug returned the next day, he didn't insist on snapping so much.

But the amazing thing is that he got the footage on the extended hard drive, got the script continuity pages together, and helped make Clint's life infinitely easier in post-production.

Script supervisors make everyone's life on set, and in post-production, that much easier. Even though Doug, at times, drove me crazy on set, he was a wonderful team player, and kind of a savant.

A man with a big heart, although I don't foresee me on set with him again, he is something of a pre-production god. In that way, I *can* see myself working with him. Anyone working with Doug should know that he's a star; you just need a little patience in dealing with him.

11

ABIGAIL YATES: ACTRESS AND ASSISTANT DIRECTOR

*I*n June of 2015, I was a woman on a mission. I had just turned the big 4-0 and was keen on getting *Letters to Daniel* made by a Studio out in Hollywood, so I was attending Film-Com (a film market, not a film festival) in Nashville. It was something of a celebration, as Pamela Turner was there with her projects, and my friends, Andrew and James, had paid for my hotel stay for my birthday.

The hotel was beautiful, and they upgraded the room to a suite. Pam and I stayed in one room, and Andrew and James stayed in the other. After dropping our things off and settling in the room, we went back down in the lobby and ordered lunch at the bar while killing time until registration opened up.

When we did register, some people recognized me from the previous year. When we went to have our picture taken with the drop banner, a woman approached us and introduced herself. She was Abigail Yates, and she asked what my project was.

When I explained that it was about getting into recovery

with bipolar disorder and achieving your wildest dreams, she opened up about the fact that she knew people who also had it. I won't say who because that's her business, and their story is not mine to tell. But she related and she had dreams of Hollywood, too.

With executives working for the likes of Focus Features, and the History Channel, we really wanted a production and distribution deal. Everybody was saying Lifetime TV, but I was steadfast in wanting a theatrical release. Part of me still harbors that desire. The Academy says a feature is any movie forty minute, or longer. It looked like *Letters to Daniel* was going to end up just shy of an hour long.

I exchanged information with Abigail and kept in touch; we fell out of touch until 2017. I hired her as actress to portray Brenda Boo, the remorseful other woman in my short romantic drama, *The Weekend*. She was amazing as a second pair of hands and never bitched once about what I asked her to do.

I would make a never-seen music video for a crappy song that the musician became a prima-donna over. I just said forget it and returned the song to him. It became clear that he wanted face time in the video, and that wasn't the vision.

Apparently, during the time Abigail and I lost touch, she had battled cancer. She was a beast. And finally, when *Letters to Daniel* was ready to go, we referred to her 2015 audition for the film. We had originally cast her as Aunt Jan. A one-scene performance (she absolutely nailed it) that she took on with dedication and relish.

Fast forward to January 2011; I asked Abigail if she would be the assistant director for *Letters to Daniel*, and she agreed.

Abigail is the real deal. If she says she's going to work on your film, then she will give you everything that she has.

A couple of days before we were to start production, I

received a message. She was sick, throwing up, and other stuff. She wasn't backing out, but she was warning me that she couldn't be on the set at 7:00 a.m. She asked for a noon call. Though I was annoyed that this was happening, I knew that she wasn't doing it on purpose. I gave her the noon call time for that first day. She got there earlier, and we got a late start at the counselor's office because she forgot that I was coming to direct the film. We were an hour behind. But, thanks to everyone, we were able to hit the ground running.

Even though the address was wrong, and I was scrambling to text everyone who was at the wrong address, or lost, things smoothed themselves out. Of the first day, only two scenes were eventually cut.

The scenes that remained from that first day were fantastic and were genius level from Mark, and all the actors involved.

During the second day, Abigail really came into her own as an assistant director. When Mark explained that he needed help, she started moving and getting people to work as a unit. She made sure that we ran on time on that second day, especially when we were locked out and huddling under the roof of the Ramada Inn Conference Center during a severe thunderstorm, and the rain poured.

Mark was afraid that our exterior scene would be rained out. But, magically, the skies cleared. It was hotter than hell, and humid, as all get out, but we got the scene.

Abigail was a commanding presence; she helped by being the asshole so that I didn't have to be. The last day, when she was on everyone about the lack of time, I thought, *I absolutely hate you. We have to get this footage.* But I really didn't hate her.

When you're working in ninety-one degree heat, being reasonable takes skill, and patience. Since heat makes me anxious, and my bipolar brain was peaking on overload on the last day, that was a lot to ask of me.

But Abigail was a champ. When Doug went down on the fourth day she rose to the occasion and stepped up to be script supervisor with Missy. Between the two of them, we cranked out scenes left and right.

We had twenty pages to get through that day. Having started in Cedar Grove Coffeehouse at 7:00 a.m., and moving to Mysti Parker's house from noon, we had until 8:00 p.m. to get through all those pages.

Abigail kept us running smoothly, for the most part. We took thirty to eat and drink. To be honest, my diet was trashed on that set. During the day, I would be so anxious that I could barely get myself to eat, or drink. I just wanted to shoot the film.

It was on day four when I thought that I would have a heart attack. There was talk of us not having two key shots in the church from the third day because the camera was hot, and it wouldn't play back.

I had a meltdown and started crying. I thought, *We've come so far and, now, the dream is dead.*

While I was doing my best Chicken Little, it fell to Missy to chill me out. She later told me that I was mean to her, but I just remember feeling desperate, and lost. Until Doug said that the shots were there, I was a nervous wreck.

Missy was amazing on set. She was the de facto fire extinguisher. While I dealt with no show, no call actors, and asshat gas station managers who originally said that I had the location and, at a moment's notice changed their minds, she kept people from distracting me from directing the film.

After that first day, we went to the motel, Abigail said that there were bugs on the pillow and asked if she could stay at my house. My parents were cool and said, "Yes."

We did tarot cards and partook of tasty meals and kept crazy hours. I was sleep-deprived, for the most part.

Abigail was a great team player. She was a hard worker and when, Mark and I needed her, she was a Godsend.

She was also cast as Pamela Turner, the third member of 3 Bitches Press. She attended the funeral scene. She was in three other scenes, but all except one was cut, which was a shame, because she was quite good.

Abigail made sure that we took breaks. She made sure that I ate when Missy was busy with another part of the film.

Building up to the shoot, there were lots of late night chats about her dreams, about putting one's hopes and dreams out into the universe and stepping out in faith. She wanted to get her acting career in gear, but she found herself stymied by financial setbacks.

I understood where she was coming from.

Letters to Daniel was born as something of a fluke. I had written my hero, and I couldn't cram my life story into one letter. The blog helped me grow stronger, and more stable, much like this book is helping me recover from the insanity that was the film.

But those letters came straight from the heart about the realities of living with, and recovering from, bipolar disorder. They demonstrated that life was not pure success, as some outside observers would have you believe. There were ups, downs, setbacks and, yes, successes.

But bipolar disorder was always there, always lurking, watching, waiting to strike when I least expected it.

In a sense, I walk a tightrope every day. I don't know if I'm going to wake up on the wrong side of the bipolar bed. Am I going to be sucked into my bed? Am I going to be filled with self-loathing? Or will I wake-up peppy, and full energy, ready to start the day?

It's often hard to be rational when I'm twisted up from the disorder. I'm anxious, and full of varying degrees of paranoia. I also find it hard to completely trust anyone.

So, while making a film with so many moving parts, I knew that would rub my bipolar all kinds of wrong ways. I also knew I could do it, though. With the right team behind me, and people there who knew what to look for during the shoot to make sure I didn't go off deep end, I knew that I could do it.

With Abigail, she was an added value player. She did more than what was asked of her. She didn't flinch where hard work was concerned. I would recommend her as a crew member in a heartbeat, and I hope to give her a meatier role to sink her teeth into. But, given that my next serious project is a television pilot in *Recovery Unplugged*, I would need to recruit her as a crew member again. Having sponsors would enable me to pay everyone, including Thomas Moore and his partner, Jay.

Recovery Unplugged is *Letters to Daniel*'s direct legacy. It combines my love of the creative arts with my passion for mental health advocacy. I already have my first sponsor signed on, and I plan on using the polished version of *Letters to Daniel* to leverage myself more sponsorships. Things look good on the horizon, and it's because of the help I receive from people like Abigail that I'm getting there.

12

THOMAS MOORE: FILMMAKER, ADVOCATE, FRIEND

I met Thomas at the 2016 Imaginarium. I was sitting on documentary panel, and Thomas was attending. It was my third go-round with Imaginarium, and it was his first. I remember sitting there and, when another guest on the panel talked about raising fifteen grand for her movie, I thought, *Not even close, honey, my movies usually cost less than a thousand a dollars. And that's being generous.* I could tell that Thomas was in the same boat.

He made his movies for very little, if anything at all. He had developed a team who was devoted to him, and his dream. Over the course of the panel, he opened up a bit, and we discovered that we had something in common. We both were diagnosed with bipolar disorder, and our connection was instantaneous.

It's hard to explain. We bi-polars tend to identify one another in a crowd. I call them psychological siblings. He's not the only one I have, but I message him almost daily, and he respects me as an artist. I think that he prefers my documentaries to my narrative films, but I always appreciate his feedback, whether I agree with him, or not. His honesty is not born out of maliciousness; it simply comes out of a desire to help.

That year, *Letters to Daniel: Awareness* won for Best Non-Genre Short Film. He won for *Incumbent*, Best Director Runner-Up. I've been shut out there since, and I can't seem to shake the runner-up moniker.

I immediately friended him on FB and messaged him that he should submit his work to AOF. He did so, and he was rewarded for his efforts.

He directed a movie called *Ruination*. It is an anti-suicide film which doesn't flinch when it comes to talking about finding a permanent decision for a temporary state of mind. It opens up discussion about how that state of mind clouds your judgment, yet it does not judge the heroine for her mental illness. It's a powerful film, and a real gut punch. I felt like it was the best film at Imaginarium 2017, hands down. However, the judges did not agree with me and awarded him with a runner-up trophy.

To which I say to them, "Shame on you." Don't get me wrong, I adore Imaginarium, and everything it has done for me, but they've made some weird calls on certain films during the recent years. That's the thing about film festivals, different directors have a taste for different things.

I attend Imaginarium primarily for the creative writing aspect. I've developed a workshop, Thriving Creatively While Coping with Serious Mental Illness. I got to teach it for the first time at Imaginarium, and I got to give again, for the second time, thanks to Shon Jason Medley and Con Nooga.

It's inspired by my part memoir, part how-to book, *Something to Believe In*. It instructs on how to thrive creatively, even in the face of severe mental illness. It differs from the documentary to a certain degree, but they make great companion pieces to one another.

Thomas and I have always been in sync about being mental health advocates. He does it with his film, *Ruination*. I'm constantly doing it through some facet of my work. People should and, if they are familiar at all with the *Letters to Daniel* brand, then they know that I've been through a lot in my life, especially if they've followed the blog or read my memoir or have seen the documentaries *Letters to Daniel: Breakdown to Bestseller* or *All in the Family*.

Something to Believe In the documentary is a look at what *Letters to Daniel* is, and what it has meant for my healing process, and career.

When Thomas admitted to me that he had bipolar disorder, I couldn't say that I was shocked, but that's what *Letters to Daniel* has done to this point. It opens up conversations with people who may not have felt comfortable doing so otherwise.

I used the memoir as an outreach, sometimes not charging for it if the person really needed to know that they weren't alone.

The year *Awareness* was playing, Thomas was new to the Imaginarium scene. He was there: Nathan Day, and his film.

Thomas is a genius. I seem to have the good luck of running into such brilliant people on the circuit. He has a really sharp eye for storytelling. In my opinion, we make a great writer(me)/director(him) team. He cut my trailer for *Letters to Daniel*. And he and his partner Jay, along with Clint, Missy, and Tim Druck (more on him later) had agreed to work with me on *Recovery Unplugged*, my mental health advocacy talk show that explores artists, their battles with mental illness, and it impacts their professional and personal lives.

I've done it as a podcast for nineteen episodes. I think I will focus on bringing sponsors on board. I'm going to AOF to find them. Finding money in an any endeavor is hard. I wish I had the trailer all cut and the sound cleaned and scored and ready to go. That way, they would have an example of my best work to date.

Thomas does great trailers! That's why I'm excited to have him on board, cutting it together. He has sixteen short films under his belt. He wants his crack at the big time, as do all of us, for the most part. The filmmaker who tells you, "I want to make a film that nobody will see, and will make zero dollars," is a liar.

I may not be driven to do this solely for the money, but I get satisfaction a story well-told. But I obviously have a drive for people to hear my voice and to take me seriously as a filmmaker. And, over the years, I've been seen as a one hit wonder, which couldn't be further from the truth.

I have almost as many produced films as I do published novels. I have twenty-three films/videos, and twenty-four published books. All the films are award-winning, and eleven of the books are Amazon bestsellers. Thirty-two are award winning scripts. I also have many more books on the way.

Thomas and I push each other. He sends me his work, and I send him mine, usually bracing for impact. I'm hopeful that he'll love *Letters to Daniel*, as he has always been supportive of my projects that involve my personal story.

Actually, he supports all of it, I just don't think he likes everything I do. But that's not a cut on him. He's honest, but he's not unkind.

Everyone who has seen *Letters to Daniel* remarked what a huge leap it was for me. I always have talent in front, but I think the top-heavy talent was provided, in no small part, to Thomas. I had Brandon X Bell, but he introduced me to Knoxville's best kept acting secrets, Megan Jones and Virginia Beld.

Maria Christian absolutely nailed the narration. But, then, I already knew that she could, and would. I had seen Megan in *Ruination* and Virginia in *Salt in the Wound*. I knew they were good actresses and, when they auditioned together, they had fantastic chemistry.

You can't force, or fake, chemistry. Either the actors have it, or they don't. Megan and Ginny and Brandon all had great chemistry, and it was a gamble putting Brandon with Virginia. What I think has been one of the more enjoyable parts of the editing process was watching Ginny's acting, (which is already good) get better in her scenes with Brandon. She is natural throughout, but especially so with Brandon.

That brings me to Brandon; he is such an open, and generous, actor. Professional. I'll steal a line from Shemar Moore when he was talking about Kristoff St. John, (Neil Winters on *The Young and the Restless*) "Brandon is the Denzel of Cleveland."

I met him through Indie Gathering, where he has been nominated for Best Supporting Actor three times. I did *Broken* with him, and he received a Best Lead Actor nomination at Hollywood Dreamz.

I have worked with Brandon on three films, and he always comes to play. He doesn't goof off. He knows when it's time to work, and when it's time to play.

Those girls, Megan and Ginny, were fantabulous! Megan was me. Anybody who really knows from during that time knows how difficult it was. I was in a constant, hellish head-space. Who I am kidding, I was in hell, and Missy was there as a constant.

I really want to wait before I talk too much about them. These actors, and few others, went above and beyond the call of duty.

Back to Thomas. I would have never met Thomas were it not for Imaginarium, even though time at the 2016 Imaginarium was bittersweet. The best thing to come out of it that year was my friendship with him.

Often times, we talk about fun stuff, serious stuff, and our hopes for our futures: the desire to really collaborate, to have the money to execute on a level we'd both be proud of. We talked about when people in our lives shit on our dreams, and we'd listen and give hope to each other when we got frustrated.

Because of #Me Too Movement, there's been a push to hire women. I had more women on my set, and I found great people to surround myself with.

When I say that I found great people, I have Indie Gathering to thank (Brandon X Bell, John Spalding, Aaron Allen, Doug Kaufman, Laura Masi Cline, and her son, Michael, Valyo Gennoff) and AOF (Mark Maness and Clint Gaige) and Imaginarium (Megan and Virginia). As I can attest to, all of these people were simply wonderful. So was Tim, who's been my friend since high school.

He likes to say he was there at the beginning of *Letters to Daniel*. The first person whom I told was Missy. It's always been Missy. God help the men who will marry us. We call each other, every day, multiple times a day. We're fixtures in one another's lives. Tim has been for a lot of things and he really, more than most people, understood what it meant for me to accomplish shooting the film.

I had told Tim, when Harold was sick and the odds were stacking up against him, I realized that I don't have forever on this earth. I realized my career, as both a writer and as a filmmaker was concerned, that the mountain wasn't going to come to Mohammed, Mohammed was going to have to go to the mountain.

Tim said, "Amy, most people have to scale the mountain. You had to level, you proved, in the end, the only thing stopping you is money."

And I said, "I did it, anyway."

"Hells, yeah!" he replied.

Thomas couldn't wait to see a final cut of the movie. And, frankly, I couldn't wait for him to see it, either.

13

JOHN SPALDING: G1NBC, AND MY
LINE PRODUCER

*J*ohn. Where do we begin with John Spalding? During the fall of 201, I co-wrote, and directed, the short romantic drama, *Broken*. I worked with Brandon Bell and Maria Christian. Brandon interviewed the cast and crew while we ate and drank (some more so than others) and recorded them for Brandon's connection in Ohio, G1NBC of Cuyahoga County.

A few months later, we all gathered together for John to interview us about our experience. He would go on to broadcast *Letters to Daniel: Breakdown to Bestseller*, *Black Gold: Trail to Standing Rock*, *Broken*, and *All in the Family* and create a page for me to blog on, sort of a continuance of the *Letters to Daniel* theme.

It's funny, ever since making the movie, I haven't felt the need to blog, but I did feel the need to tell the story of how the film got made, and John Spalding was a guardian angel. After the third representative lied to me about having twenty-thousand dollars for my project, I reached out to John and explained that I needed a producer. Well, he didn't exactly do that. He signed on as line producer and began to raise my profile all across social media. I had already done a good job, but he helped take it to another level.

He steadied a rocking ship and staunched the bleeding. He was a stabilizing force which helped me not to lose faith that, somehow, I would get it done.

He would go on to boost certain posts. He'd campaigned and promoted as hard as me, and it had been magical.

When he arrived at the hotel with his cot, he didn't complain. When one's hotel room has mold in the shower, and bugs in the bed, most people, understandably, bail. He had to buy his own towel, and replace the toilet paper. And, yet, he stayed for production and became the hardest working as far as physical labor goes person on set outside of Mark Maness. He earned the title of key grip and stepped in when our Harold Goodman no called, no showed, and no acted.

He was a natural, and led by example. Building up to the production, we were producing, and executing, the podcast/series *Recovery Unplugged.* We were interviewing independent directors, writers of all kinds, actors, and festival directors.

John deftly guided me through the opening banter, and I dove into the interviews: people like Geoffrey Calhoun, Del Weston, and filmmakers, such as Thomas Moore, actors, such as Brandon X. Bell, and Anabelle Munro. It had really flourished, and my connection to G1NBC had yielded a business partnership that is both creative and steady.

In a business that does not encourage stability, it does quite the opposite; it invites chaos into our lives. And, if you're not well-grounded with an amazing team of support around you, you will not remain anchored and tethered to your sanity.

John came along at just the right time. AOF had done a lot

to repair my self-image after the trauma I had encountered with my management team. He established a Bitcoin account for me, and a Bitcoin fundraiser.

Neither generated the kind of funds we needed, but they both contributed to spread of the brand, and the reach of people wanting to know more, and that was invaluable.

The journey to make a feature film starts as seed and, if it is nurtured and showered with hard work, grit, love, perseverance, and determination, then there is no limit as to what you can do.

And, when I messaged him a million times about fundraising, broadcasts of my films, attending festivals, or simply touching base for *Recovery Unplugged* and who is going to be on the show that week, he was (mostly) understanding.

He always had a sarcastic sense of humor, and I always give him hell about being a Browns fan. Yes, they had a good year last year but, before that, they were The Bad News Bears of the NFL. (That joke is especially for you, John.) But no one worked harder along with me than John, other than Missy, throughout the development of *Letters to Daniel* since coming aboard.

Anyone who has to handle me has to be long on patience. My mood is relatively stable, but it's not without its hiccups. That summer has been brilliant all because I had an amazing, hard-working team around me, pushing me to do my best, and raise my level of filmmaking to a professional level.

And I feel like the place where my film is falling down right now is the sound. Can't work with amateurs but, in reality, volunteers were all I could afford. No one local wanted to work for the crumbs that I could afford.

Valyo, whom I met at Indie Gathering, sprinkled his magic on it, so the sound was considerably improved. We don't have the finances, or the logistic ability, to do ADR and Foley. Our budget, while more than we've had before, was nowhere near what other folks have, and a marathon away from what a major studio has to spend on their films.

Priming the marketing pump without saturating the market is a delicate dance. As my profile rose, *Letters to Daniel* developed. All the people I would draw to my team, they had me in awe of either their talent, their hard work, or their can willingness to sacrifice comfort in the name of the project.

Intown Suites was truly a hotel of horrors: drug dealers lurking in vans, drug paraphernalia, cramped quarters, ungodly early mornings to hit the set, long days that stretched into the nights sometimes.

But no one left, and no one quit. Everybody gave their best but, then, we were in the last stages of post-production. Sound. I'd prayed that Valyo could rise to the challenge that our film represented at the moment. I will be honest and say the sound was not that great when we started out, but Valyo pulled it off.

I headed to Indie Gathering that weekend. We were only there for two nights. But I'm hoping Brandon will come for a little while and so will John. Maybe Laura and Michael, too. Actors in my movie with an Indie Gathering Connection.

John Spalding is a blue collar guy with a liberal mindset. I love that about him. He likes to tease because I take everything so literally, (I hate that.) But he has consistently supported me in my creative endeavors: broadcasting my work, supporting projects that I am passionate about.

The next step in the *Letters to Daniel* legacy *is Recovery Unplugged*. It is my dream project now, to do a television talk show that addresses mental illness in the creative community, celebrities and indie artists alike, while providing resources to the independent artist they might not otherwise have.

I know that it's hard to launch a talk show without a major platform, but Upliftv has expressed interest in it, and Clint

Gaige wants to film an entire season in one week. So I will be on the hunt tomorrow for sponsorships once again. And will look for them at Indie Gathering. I'll have to hit the ground running. But I plan on lining up meetings when I get there.

Recovery Unplugged has nineteen proof of concept podcast episodes. I hope to parlay that into some interest.

And I really have to build my team. I have a camera; I have sound equipment. Need three cameras, have one, will look into getting another two. We have to film the entire first season to get sponsorships from the television network, and that means finding funding for the first ten episodes. It will be a challenge, but we are up to it. I have a crowdfunding campaign in my head, and am excited, to say the least. I will definitely recruit John Spalding.

Because John Spalding is awesome-sauce, I would have never been able to make *Letters to Daniel* without him.

His cool head in pre-production helped to keep from hanging on by my fingernails. And, by him helping Mark out the way he did during his time on set, it saved the movie from falling apart. He was beast onset, and a terrific actor.

He was a natural in front of the camera. But, to be fair I saw him in the comedy, *In Production*, where he was a hilarious pot-dealing Jewish man. For *Letters to Daniel*, he represented Harold Goodman (Missy's father) very well.

I'm going to ask him to help with crowdfunding for *Recovery Unplugged*. I think after the kind of year I just had at AOF, my network will be larger.

Recovery Unplugged is a passion project, just like *Letters to Daniel* was, and it extends my advocacy work. I can impact a group that I think is very stigmatized, and that is Christian viewers. The church is notorious for stigmatizing people with mental illness and doing them a disservice by telling them that God doesn't give you more than you can handle, or to just pray it away.

While those organizations are well-intentioned, mental illness doesn't work that way. I believe in God, but I believe that God gave us psychiatrists and therapists as healers, and He gave us the good sense to know when to use them.

Not that faith in God, or a strong spiritual core, is a negative thing; it's not. Prayer and mindful meditation are powerful tools you can use to manage your illness and to guide you to not just to survive, but also to thrive.

I'm living proof that recovery is possible, and dreams really do come true, and John is one the reasons for that. He doesn't know how much I really appreciate all of his hard work and, hopefully, on the next project, I can pay him what he's worth and put him in a much nicer hotel, or at least a clean one, where he doesn't have to buy toilet paper, or pay for his towels to be cleaned.

John, in case you're reading this, I adore you, even though you tease me and piss me off sometimes. Here's to a long creative partnership; may it be fruitful, and profitable.

14

TIM DRUCK: JACK OF ALL TRADES, AND ALWAYS THERE WHEN I NEED HIM

I have known Tim since I was fifteen years old. That's close to thirty years. We attended the same high school, Louisville Central High School, for two years: him for the computer technology magnet, me for the law magnet. While he would go on to use his knowledge gained through his time at Central to apply his experience in real life venues, such as the Navy, and by parlaying his knowledge into a career as a graphic artist as well.

Tim was a member of the band LAME, and directed the documentary #allweknowislame, an account of how their seventeen-year-old drummer experienced a catastrophic car accident and was hooked up to life support. The rest of the band were told that, if he lived, he would be a vegetable. The accident took place October of 2014. Evan would walk out of the hospital under his own power two months later, and he had his first practice with the band in January 2015.

They would have a triumphant concert in 2016 at Diamonds, but would disband in 2018. This devastated Tim and, since he struggles with mood stability, (undiagnosed. I observed by his actions, and emotional posts, on Facebook, and by just being his friend) it took him a while for him to get over the breakup. Alex and Evan are considerably younger than Tim, and they have moved on to create music without him.

This was especially hurtful to Tim. On top of which, he was busting his ass at the Hookah Lounge with no creative outlet. His brother passed away due to a heroin addiction. I really wondered if Tim was going to be any help at all.

That much grief can be hard for anyone, add possible undiagnosed mental illness to the mix, and it can really pull you under. As time grew closer to production, I would tap Tim on the FB shoulder from time to time. He was totally down, but he answered, (most of the time). Like I said, it was understandable and, when it got to be got to be go time, Tim was there for us.

Was I always happy with him during filming? Well, to be totally honest, no. He ducked out early the first day to help someone else at the Louisville Palace, (however, it was a paying gig, and how do you really compete with that). Then, Sundays were a non-factor because he was exhausted by that point. He was working until three in the morning and then showing up on set at seven. Finally, on the fourth day, he was well rested, and he perked up. And, on Tuesday, he lived up to his nickname, Tim "the Mayor" Druck by pulling a location out of his ass and saving the whole production.

Many thanks to Hippyhead, and OG Auto. They gave us amazing shots, and some of them weren't even used. I could have put my foot down and had two more scenes added, and an extra song at the end. That would have pushed me to seventy minutes, but I think it would have killed the quality of the finished product, so we have a sixty-one-minute feature which is eligible for the Emmys.

With possible distribution from Upliftv, that's a distinct possibility. I am patiently waiting for Del to send me notes and emails and contacts to various international distributors, including those getting *Letters to Daniel* on airlines.

I was so stoked; my greatest hope was to have a small volunteer army with me to help run the Free Your Mind International Film Festival. Although, with people's work schedules, that proved to be interesting.

I was so thrilled that *Letters to Daniel* seemed set to explode. People mocked, and underestimated, me for keeping at the *LtD* pump for six years, and it's so nice to be able to prove those people wrong and not feel like I have to punish them for it.

I went to AOF and attended a Life Council Panel and heard Dr. Bob Goldman, Susan Stafford, Lee Broda, and Magie Cook speak. They are amazing individuals, and humanitarians.

Magie Cook was an orphan who lived in poverty in Mexico and, with only a knife to hunt for and feed her sixty-eight siblings. She was homeless and was given an $800.00 gift which she parlayed into a multi-million-dollar salsa business she sold to Campbell's Soup for over two-hundred million dollars.

She is humble, sweet and, when I asked if I could send her my scripts, she said, "Yes"! Her dream is to be an actress. I also hope to be a part of that someday.

One final note about Magie: when her kids were kidnapped and sold into human trafficking, she, her brother, and Mexican Federalies went after them. As Magie and her brother waited with the kids in a hotel room, her with a .38 special and her brother with a shotgun aimed at the door, she was prepared to give her life for those kids.

Those are the kind of people whom you normally meet at AOF; just meeting her was a gift. She touched my soul with her words and her genuine, authentic self. I've met many people along the way at AOF who have changed my life. I hope that Tim gets to come and experience it. And I also hope that Missy comes for all ten days. I want them to shower her with the kind of love they have me.

Tim is always someone whom I can count on. Whether it's for an impromptu guerilla photo shoot because Del Weston has asked for twenty-thirty quality photos, or it's coming up with a location in the 11th hour, he's a cool cat.

But, like me, he's vulnerable to his mind, and his emotions, betraying him. He's a sensitive soul, and a political activist. He has a keen insight regarding injustice against others. And, when he puts pen to paper, he is quite eloquent, and fiery.

However, in his heart of hearts, he's a musician, a bass player. He recently moved on and formed another band, Pulse. His passion is music and, when his soul is being fed, he couldn't be happier.

He dreams of finishing a documentary and filming mine and Missy's award-winning short script, *Rain Down on Me*.

He often gets in his own way and, with a daughter heading into her senior year of high school, he's got her college years on his mind.

Yet he made time for *Letters to Daniel*. In fact, his whole family did. Abby and Caitlyn were there for acting on day two, and Caitlyn was there five out of the six days of filming, slating, and doing makeup.

Tim labored for simply meals and IMDb credits. He wanted this so badly for me and, when I finally executed it, we both found ourselves without words.

What do you say to someone who has taken the journey with you and you complete that chapter of the story with them; there's something to be said for that. Tim exited my life in high school and wandered back into it after my first books were published.

We started talking on FB and reconnected. The odd thing is I remembered him as this kid, whose energy rubbed me the wrong way, and he got on my nerves. Tim still has the unique capacity to drive absolutely insane but, most of the time, he's good.

But, at the same time, he's got the largest heart and is something of a humanitarian. He is often an ear for me to bend late at night, or during the wee hours of the morning.

Talking to Tim about art is a lot of fun. I often get frustrated with him because he has a lot of raw talent, which just needs refining. He often gets so close to really going somewhere, then, his mindset sometimes causes him to self-destruct. But when he loves, he loves big, and you won't find a more loyal friend.

His family is wonderful, too. Abby keeps his butt in line, and his spirit lifted. And he said he lucked out because he got the coolest kid.

Tim is, at times, the perpetual big brother/just one of the guys. He vacillates between the two and, depending on the day, and depending on what he's going through, he could be either one, sometimes both.

But, despite all my frustrations with Tim, he is someone you want in your corner. We renewed our friendship in 2012, and it's been going strong ever since. He played at a book signing with Lame, where the cops threatened to end the signing if they didn't cool it. They also played at a place where food I bought for the room, and it got eaten by the Stan Lee crowd.

I was never reimbursed and, I won't mention the convention because they're shady, and I have no desire to welcome that chaos back into my life. They are like cockroaches, they'll never be extinct but, if I keep a good can of Raid nearby, then I should be fine.

I only really want to spread some love, and each of my regular festivals provide something different. Imaginarium is becoming less of a writing convention, and more of a comic-con. I understand that. Stephen is looking at things from a business angle. Imaginarium is intimate, and more of a writers' venue than a filmmakers'.

In 2019, there were more films, and there were lots of local entries including three podcast *Recovery Unplugged* interviews. But the class of the field in short films were Thomas Moore's *A Lady's Reckoning* in the shorts, and Mark Maness' *It Knows* in features.

We shall see what the festival reflects come the night of the awards banquet. You never can tell.

Tim attended Imaginarium in 2015, and Lame rocked the house. He won Best Documentary for #allweknowislame. He pitched an agent, and she accepted. When he won Best Documentary, he jumped into the pool while everyone from the convention lined up against the window to watch take off his shoes cannonball into the water.

The fact that his cohorts in the band started creating without him had devastated him. All the while, he had to deal with his brother's death.

Missy was the set mother. Doug would collapse in exhaustion, and trauma from his past would rear its ugly head. Sobbing in Missy's arms, she made sure that he had a cool place to lie down.

When we shot the scene of me sleeping, and my dad coming to tell me that Missy's dad had died, it got to Tim. He found out about his brother's overdose after someone banged on the door.

I was so wrapped up in filming that it was left to Missy to

comfort him and to deal with the pain it had brought up for her. I didn't notice, until after the series of scenes addressing her father's death, that there were tears in her eyes.

Good director, but not so great a friend. Missy said that I was the queen of the side eye every time she had a suggestion. That was my fear. When I get on a set, I tend to get tunnel vision. I was able to communicate well with Mark, but I had worked solo so much during pre-production. From devising the shot list, to gathering the cast, (which Missy vetted) we chose Megan and Ginny together.

After comforting one another, they didn't miss a beat. When we were finished, he told me how proud of me he was. And, when I told Mark that I was getting the Founder's Award for my body of work, I also mentioned that everyone at the festival had managed to make a film. I realized that my career was like the mountain. It wasn't going to come to me, I was going to have to go to it.

He said to me, "Amy, most people have to climb the mountain. You had to level it."

And, thanks to friends in my life like him, I was able to do so.

15

JUSTIN & JULES: THE TAG TEAM SOUND TEAM

*O*h, the trials and tribulations of hiring sound people. Sound people generally don't work for IMDb credits, shelter, and even meals on set. The good ones are expensive because, let's face it, they can be.

It is everyone's goal in independent film to make a salary, or a fair wage. But let's be realistic, some of us don't have the means by which to pay everyone what they're worth. Sometimes, the best we can do is a little gas money, food, and an IMDb credit. And, on rare occasions, we can house our casts and crew.

I'll be honest, our backs were up against a wall. We were a month out, and we had no one. Then, Missy's cousin, Justin Simmons, a total doll, said that he would help us. Justin also mentioned that he was nervous because he had never worked with equipment professionally, but he had been shown the ropes during high school.

Although his lack of experience would prove somewhat

problematic during past, the fact remains that, if he hadn't said, "Yes," then we would have had no one on the first three days.

Justin came every day that he could and always had a great all in, team player attitude. He never complained, and he worked his ass off.

When called upon to act, he rose to the occasion. Unfortunately for him, and for us, the scene was cut. But, for the record, Justin made for a great man high on drugs, confronting the lead characters.

It was a total pleasure to work with him. He was always on time, and ready to work. He did what was asked of him, and with zero sense of entitlement.

Given that he was twenty-one years old, and had no ego to speak of, it really spoke to his character. He bonded with Tim's daughter, Caitlyn, and threw Mark for loop when he had her do his eyeshadow.

Even though he was only with us for four out of the six days, he always ready to go the distance. His inexperience at boom placement notwithstanding, he got us good enough sound to produce the scenes that we needed, and Valyo had worked miracles in the tougher spots. I simply couldn't wait to hear all though Valyo had put together.

Justin is such a sweet kid. I couldn't wait for him to see the final product, to feel the accomplishment of a job well done. He tried his damndest and, because he was willing to work for free, we had sound, period.

Feedback from other filmmakers included harsh remarks about the sound, but Valyo had done amazing things. And, from the way Clint and Mark talked, the sound was an unmitigated disaster. I had thought my movie was ruined. But, when I watched the film, I was relieved.

And there's been a lot of pressure for ADR, and Foley, with

a few of the scenes. And, frankly, it's not in the budget. Some had a few issues with certain spots in the editing. I respectfully disagree with that. I think Clint did a masterful job with the editing, and I was in tears at the finish.

2019 had been a big year for me. It marked my twentieth year in recovery. AOF handed me the keys to a brand-new festival, the Free Your Mind International Film, and Screenwriting Competition. They were footing the bill. Since I was the director, I chose the projects, I made the rules, and I chose the winners. The festival's mission is to serve artists with mental illness, and social disorders, who are healing themselves through their art.

When they handed the keys to the festival over to me, I was flabbergasted. Running a festival, from what I've seen, is hard, thankless work. People attack you when you don't choose their script/art/film and, when they don't win, they say things like, "They only award their friends."

I had to admit, I was not looking forward to that, but I was looking forward to affording other people like me the opportunity to change their lives. Because AOF did that, it seemed that I was miles away from that scared little girl who attended AOF in 2016.

Megafest is a festival for everyone. When I interviewed Del, he said this about his festival, "So many times, we hear 'no' in our lives, AOF strives to be the festival to say 'yes.'"

I really want my *Letters to Daniel* team to experience the love that is AOF. And the idea that I can be a cog in that wheel is tremendously exciting.

Other festivals are wonderful, but AOF is King, and Del and Theresa are mentors that don't come along every day. They take you into their embrace and say, "Let me water you with love and encouragement, provide you with opportunities for you to seek out, and enable you to connect with other artists, filmmakers, writers, composers, and actors to create future collaborations with."

And they do it on a level that keeps you pushing, even the face of setbacks. *Letters to Daniel* has been a thing for six years. First, as a blog, where I processed my everyday life with bipolar disorder, and shared my memoirs.

With each incarnation of the project, it grew and expanded in popularity. With each setback to the film, that meant time to lick my wounds, pick up the pieces, get back up, and keep pushing.

Jules, again while the results on her efforts on sound were less than satisfactory, the fact remains that, had she not volunteered, we would have been up a shit creek. She knew where to place the boom perfectly. Her experience with an h4n zoom pro was much less proficient.

But, as I've said, the sound is good enough that Valyo can work with it and salvage it. Jules, as far as attitude was a bit much. She rubbed an actress and her son the wrong way. Costing me much needed on set help.

As far as the work goes, she was an incredibly hard worker. She, along with the other women on the set, worked alongside Mark where the physical labor was concerned. She was just a real workhorse and, like I said, almost every one of my crew members ticked me off at some point.

It wasn't their fault really, the heat, the stress, and the monumental task we were taking on all conspired to rub my bipolar disorder the wrong way. Apparently, I was especially hard on Missy and, at times, she felt like I was shutting her out of the creative process.

Since I tend to get tunnel vision when directing, if I

perceive I am in charge, collaborating with another director can be difficult. Fortunately, I collaborated well with Mark.

Thomas viewed my film and proceeded to tell me what he thought was wrong with it. Some valid points were made, and others were good food for thought. Then, he then said what he liked, all of it with a grain of salt. Those were good words to take with me into my next project.

Amy Wade, 2016 AOF Rising Star, absolutely loved it; she got very emotional. "You're going to be an in-demand filmmaker," she told me.

Bob Messinger (a screenwriter/producer) and his daughter (who struggles with bipolar disorder) watched it. Bob had a few notes, all good food for thought, and his daughter was very moved.

Amy Wade also struggles with bipolar disorder. Bob and Thomas gave great feedback to improve my filmmaking skills.

But it was Amy's and Bob's daughters' responses that move me. They both have bipolar disorder, and they felt like they were seeing themselves. That's what filmmakers live for. And, since I laid my soul bare in this film, it moves me when the viewer connects in such a raw and real way.

That's the whole reason why I made it, so that people like me don't feel so alone in this world, so that caregivers know how much I love them, and educate the ignorant or people who stigmatize the mentally ill.

It's hard to believe that *Letters to Daniel* was born as an open fan letter to my favorite actor. About halfway through the letter, I realized that I had created a platform and chose to tell my memoirs.

Today, I called Daniel Craig's attorney to attempt to get my film to him. Gatekeepers in Hollywood are notoriously hard to get through. But I hope a well written letter and the film will move them enough to tell him about and send him the link.

Shortly before filming, Omaze offered the experience of meeting Daniel Craig and touring Pinewood Studios, where they filmed the James Bond movies. I entered it multiple times. We were two days from the announcement of the winner. I tried not to think about it because the chance of me winning such a sweepstakes was astronomically stacked against me.

But I wanted to win. I wanted to be able to meet Daniel, face-to-face, and tell him how much his work has impacted my own, and how much his work has impacted me during my recovery. I'm fond of saying that Maurice Benard, with his advocacy, got me into treatment. While Daniel's work inspires my art, it ultimately keeps me there, even when I get tired of the medications and the therapy. I am firmly and acutely aware that my bipolar disorder will never "go away," that I will always need therapy and guidance from a psychiatrist.

My writing is instrumental in keeping me sane. Filming and directing, though I love it, tests me. Pre-production and filming causes expansion in my mood and threatens my stability because of all the stress that comes along with it.

But writing and editing are the opposite, completely cathartic and, after I finish writing something, it's like my spirit has been scrubbed of all the stress.

Jules and Justin frustrated me in post because of their inexperience with the equipment, but I still love both of them to bits. Without them, there would be no dream come true. Without them, there is never a starting day of production. There are no sound files, period, to send to my editor extraordinaire.

People who have harshly criticized the film say that it's like Teflon skin. I know the reality of the situation and, although my sound wasn't perfect, Valyo made it consistent. There was no voice over blasting, and no impossible to hear actress. And, on top of that, there is absolutely gorgeous music that adds to emotion of the movie which is already packed with emotion.

While at AOF, last week was incredible. When I met with Del to discuss distribution, he laid out a plan that included airlines, and other international channels. For DVD, they suggested approaching NAMI for that deal, as well as ParablesTV (Roku), Upliftv, (cable and satellite TV) and a one-time online screening on G1NBC.com. We knew that, if we aired on television first, then we could still be eligible for Emmys.

And, without Jules and Justin, skilled or not, none of the above even had a chance of happening. Will I use them again on sound again? Doubtful. But would I work them in other capacities, within a heartbeat.

In the grand scheme of things, this project which I had been harboring in my heart for six years had finally come to fruition. *Letters to Daniel* was my baby, my passion project. And, by bringing all my knowledge, all my connections, all my cash, and all my talents to bear upon it, I, along with Missy, and my entire cast and crew, manifested *Letters to Daniel* into existence. Not many people can say that they have done that, and I will be forever grateful to everyone who made it possible

16

BRANDON X BELL: THE DENZEL WASHINGTON OF CLEVELAND

*J*n 2016, I attended the Indie Gathering for the third year in row. It was there I would meet nominated actor for *Cleveland Allegories*, Brandon X Bell. Did I watch the film at Indie Gathering? Admittedly, no. I don't actually view too many films at film festivals. The bipolar disorder makes it hard for me to concentrate on the narrative.

That's not to say that Brandon didn't make an impact on me. He is the kind of individual whose warmth, charm, and genuine charisma fills any room up that he's in. And that's what got him invited to submit his reel for a role in *Broken*, a short romantic drama that addressed PTSD in veterans and sexual assault victims.

I impressed him at Indie Gathering with my multiple wins across screenplay and film categories. He impressed me and endeared himself to me with his gratitude and grace in defeat, and in his joy, for the man who'd won.

This business is filled with cutthroat individuals, who will just as soon block your success, cheer for your downfall, or even lie to you and rip you off. Brandon encompasses none of those things. His pet project is *The Connected*, a Cleveland-based web series where is portrays the head of a mafioso type family.

He endeavors through the production to hire Cleveland-based talent, and he has the right network to do it. He can make announcement on FB, and people come. He struggles at times because people abandon the production, and he is forced to scramble. But, then, that's the daily reality of indie film.

Brandon is a workhorse. You can ask him to act out the phone book, and he'd likely win an award.

I only watched *Cleveland Allegories* once I returned home. I loved his performance.

Missy wanted to see more. She said, "Now that we've seen his best Sam Jackson, let's see what else he can do."

I agreed, but the reason I wanted him to be the romantic lead in my film was because of one quiet scene where he's sitting on a bench with the lead actress. I thought, *Hey, there's something special there.*

We sent him the script and told him to self-tape two contrasting scenes for an audition. I promptly put it out of my mind and headed to Monrovia, CA for the 2016 AOF.

During one of the seminars, his video audition popped through on Messenger. I couldn't wait to get back to my room and watch it. I was out for hours. One keeps crazy hours at festivals, especially events on the West coast. When I finally got to a place where I could watch it, I was simply blown away.

Brandon has a way about him that is very natural. He comes off as authentic and really shines in front of the camera. I couldn't wait to work with him. What I learned during the fall of 2016 was that I had hit the jackpot when it came to the quality of the human being I had found for a muse. I could write for Brandon forever, if that was what he wanted. First and foremost, he's a father, and a husband. He's been through a lot, and he's just so damn lovable.

What you'll see in this business is that there is a lot of ego to go around. There are actors who are fussy about how they're lit, if they're in the shot, and will be belligerent and hold up production.

There are actors who will challenge you on every front and make production a living hell. On our first film, the lead actress constantly cursed. Though the script called for it, she flubbed it every single time, costing me time and money. To make matters worse, she and the supporting actor were not "off book."

Brandon has no ego when it comes to acting. He is an open, and generous, actor. He gives his best for each take. He doesn't hoard his energy, or his performances; he's completely there for his scene partner. I am in creative love with Brandon.

Just so we could work with him, we expanded the role of Patrick; we took dramatic license and made Patrick Missy's boyfriend. In reality, Patrick was a skinny, white, blonde haired kid in his early twenties.

When you view the film, you will see that Brandon is a six foot three black man in his early thirties. He had six scenes. All six made the cut. He never once asked, "Am I in the shot?" He never once complained that he wasn't "feeling it," and he was one to help Mark with the physical labor.

If you are casting a film, and you need a versatile, uber-talented actor, get in touch with me and I'll put you in contact with him.

We were filming on the third day at Messiah Trinity Church, and thirty some odd screaming brats were making it difficult to get the shot. To make matters worse, an actor totally no called, no showed. Just when I thought that my sanity was going to give, Brandon stepped outside and said, "Tornado sirens are going off, Amy."

I thought, *WTF? What else is going to happen?*

You shouldn't ask such a question. If you do, you're simply tempting fate on an indie film set. And, that night, the camera started overheating, so playback wouldn't work. I wouldn't know well into the next day if we got the two pivotal shots that we absolutely needed.

On the fourth day, we arrived at the Cedar Grove Coffee House, and only John Spalding, and the women on the crew, were helping Mark. Everyone was tired. Exhausted. And, by that time, they were running on caffeine and adrenaline. My nerves were totally shot and, when Mark wasn't comfortable with whether or not we had the scenes, I had a mini-meltdown.

Poor Missy, the set mother, and Producer Extraordinaire, had to keep me from losing my shit altogether. Somehow, the superhero caregiver she is, she was able to calm me down.

I really wish I had been better about collaborating with her on *Letters to Daniel*, because without her on set, I couldn't have executed a fraction of what I did.

She did everything from put out personnel fires to making sure that things ran smoothly. She even made a decision that I didn't like, but decided to live with, because I didn't have it in me to fight her on it. It turned out to be a great decision; (That's why she's the producer with capital P). It reinvigorated a very tired cast and crew, made Mark much happier, as it meant that he was going home two days early.

Not only that there was an emergency at the dumpster fire of motel that I had unwittingly stuck my ever valiant cast and crew in, the manager in an attempt to shake me down, had called and threatened me.

We called the 800 number, and they told us that we had

one room until the 29th. The manager went to my script supervisor's room hammered on the door, threatened him with physical violence, threatened to call the cops on him, and threatened to physically throw him out of the hotel.

Doug is a guy who can handle himself but, as he said, "I can handle one, but I don't how many friends he's got."

So, for the last night, Doug slept on my couch. It was interesting, to say the least, but he was not the only actor who took refuge there that week.

Anna-Maria slept on the couch for two nights, and Abigail was at the house for the week.

I adore my cast and crew. There was zero ego on that set, everyone believed in mine and Missy's vision, and they all worked diligently to attain it. Brandon was a true leader.

I think he's just a natural born leader. He works to give you exactly what you need, without any bullshit. I've been entangled with bullshit artists before, and it's no fun.

They like to get their hooks into you and, when you try to extract yourself, they pull and tear. The pain of breaking the connection is worth it, though. You may be left with wounds that take a long time to heal but, if I hadn't rid myself of the bullshit artists, I would have never been free to discover some like Brandon.

I love working with him. I usually cast him as complicated, or straight out good. But, for our next film together, a martial arts drama, he will play the heavy. It will star Farid Jamal Khan, Jan Kubenka, and Megan Jones. I want Brandon to feel absolutely free to define his character. I want people love to hate him. I want him to win all kinds of awards. But then, of course, I want all my actors to.

We had a great family atmosphere on the set of *Letters to*

Daniel the way it all went down. Even when it was rough, we stuck together like glue, and didn't turn on each other.

I'm not one to get religious but, after all me and Missy went through to make this film happen, it feels like once we said, "Dammit we're doing it ourselves." Things started to move so that we could.

I worry about things in the film: the *Avengers* poster, he cellphone, the *MIB* International standee. I pray the audience listens to the message and doesn't nitpick. I loved what my film looked like, especially after Valyo had finished it.

We worked so hard to level up with this film: from Mark, to the sound equipment, to the editor and actors, and the crew. Everyone was just a dream to work with.

Maria Christian, and Brandon, last worked on the same film in the fall of 2016. It was nice that they both worked on *Letters*, even though they were never on set together.

In short, Brandon is what you call an added value player. He brings something special to each project that he does. He did it on *Broken*, where he was nominated for Best Lead Actor-Short at Hollywood Dreamz, and again for Outstanding Performance by A Cast-Short for the same film.

It is my hope that, when I take *Letters to Daniel* to AOF, it will receive numerous nominations. It has been quite the journey to bring it this far. And, so far, everyone who's seen it has kind words for Brandon's performance and what was special about it was that Ginny was even better, and she was already pretty great.

17

MARIA CHRISTIAN: THE VOICE TALENT

I initially met Maria in 2015, when she auditioned for the part of *Missy in Letters to Daniel*. She was excellent. The only thing was that Kelsey Walsh auditioned and had that indefinable quality which, for a time, made her the perfect Missy. As time would pass, she would bow out (as it will sometimes happen) of the production, forcing us back to square one.

As I've already said, I'd already worked with her on *Broken*, but she is an exceptional voice actress as well. I proceeded to use her on *Black Gold: The Trail to Standing Rock* and *All in the Family*.

So, when it came time to cast a narrator for *Letters to Daniel*, I turned to her once again. And what a decision! She executed it flawlessly, and helped bring a dimension of my film to life, without it intruding on the rest of film.

Now, there is acting for the camera, and voice acting. Some can do both, but they're both very different skillsets. While Megan is an amazing actress, at the time of casting, she was an unknown quantity where it came to narrating a movie. I had worked with Maria both in front of, and behind, the camera as narrator. And, as far as voice actresses go, she is one of the best.

It was cost effective. We would have never been able to afford so much time in the recording studio otherwise.

Missy and I discovered Maria during an open casting call in Louisville, KY for *Letters to Daniel* in 2015. She had been a finalist for the part of Missy. She travelled all the way from Big Stone Gap, Virginia to audition for us. She even brought her son along.

She was very good, but Kelsey was the front runner from day one. We didn't cast her initially. Kelsey was local to Louisville. Less expense, plus she had that indefinable quality that we were looking for in the Missy character.

So we moved along.

Fast forward to the fall of 2016, and we are casting for the short, *Broken*. Maria auditioned and absolutely nailed it!

I'll be honest, since I started making films, (since 2014) I've been spoiled by the acting talent afforded to me for my shorts and features. But I've also had my share of divas and drunks (pre-2014).

Maria, when I met her, was striking out on her acting path. She had been pigeon-holed as a maid, or prostitute, so *Broken* afforded her the opportunity to stretch her wings. In *Broken*, she was the female lead and played the homeless art curator struggling from PTSD from when she was raped as a child by her father.

She was exquisite and nuanced in her performance and the other half of the reason why *Broken* was nominated for Outstanding Performance by A Cast-Short.

I got to know Maria a little bit over the course of the weekend when we shot *Broken*. I found out that she was a super-fan who worked for, GISHWHES, a non-profit founded by Mischa Collins of *Supernatural* fame. And that acting wasn't something her culture really viewed as a viable option as a career. Both her husband and son supported her dream, but her agent typecast her by her race. Maria has an ethnically ambiguous look: Indigenous, Asian, Caucasian, Hispanic. Truly, any role is within her grasp. Her agent sent her out as voice talent for animation. And, locally, she often nabs roles in true crime series and shows like *American Haunting.*

After *Broken,* she made some life decisions that were not conducive to her traveling and acting. She remains active in the Virginia area, and I have gone on to employ her as voice talent for several movies.

Maria saved our butts on *Letters to Daniel.* Voice acting is very different than acting in front of the camera. Like I said, not everyone can do it. More than that, not everyone can do it well.

Maria is one of those rare talents who can do it, and do it well.

When I listened to her performance with the narration, it brought tears to my eyes. When you have a vision of something for four years, you desperately hope for everything to play out as you had planned; you need an arsenal of exceptional actors and actresses.

Everyone who sees the movie doesn't always understand my choice to use a narrator at all. My recovery is very much entwined in the *Letters to Daniel* project, and the project originated with a Dear Diary, or Dear God fashion relating my memoirs, and my daily life, with bipolar disorder. It did not take long for my blog to generate positive feedback.

That's not to say it wasn't without its detractors. There were two individuals who accused me of being delusional and believing Daniel Craig was going to leave his wife and come to Kentucky, *as if*! He doesn't even know that I'm alive, let alone know about the blog. He knows absolutely nothing about my *Letters to Daniel* project, or the many incarnations it's had on its way to being a fully produced feature film.

Another individual, the crazy jealous wife of an ex-boyfriend, saw fit to call me a liar, and a fraud, in the comments section. I guess it's true what they say, you'll know that you've attained some level of success when the haters come out of the woodwork.

It's kind of like that at Indie Gathering. I've attained a level of success there. Over the five years, (six festivals) Missy and I have won fifty-seven awards there. The reaction of the audience is always twofold: they gasp when they are impressed, but they grumble when something strikes the wrong chord.

It doesn't really bother me. We've done the work, and we've put in the time. Generally, there is only love at Indie Gathering, especially from the regulars, as well as Ray and Kristina. They are regular supporters of mine and Missy's work.

My philosophy of life is, Go where the love is. And love is in abundance at AOF, Megafest, and the International Indie Gathering. Logistically, those are my automatic festivals, whether I win, (TIG) or am nominated, (AOF) or not, I just get my ass over to them.

Kristina and Ray gave me my first chance to win a trophy. I always wanted trophies, but I never got one until 2014. I had won medals, ribbons, certificates, plaques, everything that you can win, except for a trophy. That's why the Fright Night Film Festival win felt, well, a little hollow.

That festival is now defunct. It imploded, spectacularly, in 2017, and it never quite recovered. But the truth about that festival is that it never cared about its filmmakers, or their screenwriters. And the vendors they couldn't have given two shits about them.

I'm not speaking out of turn, as all of this is public record. But they're cockroaches, they will infest some other poor community and prey on desperate artists, and authors, wanting to make a name for themselves.

They were strictly pay for play, a lot of businesses are like that. But I ultimately thank them for the experience they gave me. When I attended the festival, I sold massive amounts of books. I cut my teeth on how to start stepping out of my box. And, hey, a win's a win. Well, not exactly. When the festival organizer tells you, "Just because I give you an award doesn't mean that I think your script, or film, is good," then you know you're headed for a world of hurt.

But, without them, there would have not been the shady agent who freed me of them. The one good thing that agent did was encourage me to go all in at AOF Megafest, and Action On Film quite simply changed my life.

There are people who complain that it's expensive, but your badges get you into all the incredible films, and the sensational seminars, such as the Creator's Brunch and the Writer's Gathering. There are also killer after parties, opportunities to sell your movie, and you can network with producers, and filmmakers, to see your script produced.

People say that I don't make enough money. I tell them, "Tough shit." I get less than $800.00 a month in disability, and I've managed to make it all four years that my work was accepted. I've managed to find amazing people to work with, who helped me bring my film which I labored to bring to fruition for four years. Until I just took the bull by the horns and manifested that shit.

With Aaron Allen signing on as an executive producer, he managed through his contacts, and mine, to raise $2,100.00 of the 6,000.00 budget. Missy promised two things about the summer of 2019: one, that we would make *Letters to Daniel* and, two, that I would get out to AOF. As always, Missy was good to her word.

It was my best year at AOF to date: five writing awards and one finalist across five festivals, and two film awards, one being my first award for directing and another being for my body of work. It was truly an out of body experience.

Not only that, but I also put into motion a martial arts drama with Bob Messinger, and two great upcoming action stars, Farid Jamal Khan and Jan Kubenka. Missy was producing. We even had a stunt coordinator signed on. And several avenues of distribution opened up to *Letters to Daniel*!

It was my best year ever. I had a wonderful time. Every year is like Disney World for me, regardless of whether I win, or lose. On top of all that, five producers asked me for my work.

I go to smaller festivals, too, ones with heart. Indie Gathering has fantastic seminars, a family community, and they truly draw world class screenwriting talent to their competition. I'm proud to be a regular attendee, even though I had to spend twenty hours on a bus to get up there for two nights. (Ten hours there, ten hours back.) It was worth it.

For the first time, people came to me, not the other way around. Winning twelve awards will do that for you. But, then, I've been coming and winning like that since 2014. I know that I hold the record, and I work hard to maintain it. But what I really want from Indie Gathering are the belt, and the hall of fame award. It won't be the end of the world if I never receive those, however, because of the talent agent we met there in 2015, the golden-voiced Maria Christian. For that, and so many other reasons, I will always love Indie Gathering.

18

THE STARS: MEGAN JONES AND VIRGINIA BELD

The hunt for who would play Amy and Missy in *Letters to Daniel* would start, in earnest, in January of 2019. When Kelsey bowed out, and Kat kind of just "disappeared" from the radar, we were left without viable options to carry our film.

It was hard bringing in new people. We had labored for so long under the belief that we had our leads. But things happen and, therefore, we started the screening process all over again. Two of the original cast from 2015 made it to shooting.

As we hunted for our Missy and Amy, I reached out to everyone I knew. We had one girl who made for a promising Missy, but our hunt for Amy proved fruitless. I was looking for the quality in the girl that made her edgy, sick, unbearable, but still sympathetic. And, while some girls had some of the qualities, no one girl proved to have them all.

I reached out to Maria because I had worked well with her, both in front of, and behind the camera. She made it clear that her duties as a wife and mother were consuming her time, and she could not travel to Kentucky to star in *Letters to Daniel*. Her work as a narrator on *Black Gold* and *All in the Family* established her as my go to girl voice over work. I had to find the Amy to match her talent, someone who could portray both the stable and the sick Amy.

That's when I asked Thomas Moore to put me in touch with two actresses whom he had worked with, Megan Jones and Virginia Beld. Both of them kind of grabbed my attention. Thomas likes her actresses overwrought, and that's okay. It works for his films. He usually does an obscenely large amount of takes. He says that he's gone as high as twenty-three takes.

I can't wrap my head around that. Three takes, maximum. Sometimes four. And, usually more than that, actors on my set tend to get worse instead of better. Thomas is a fucking brilliant director, but we have differing philosophies regarding key areas.

He did me a solid by prepping with the girls before they came down here to audition. That's another thing. When Megan sent her tape in as Amy, I knew, immediately, that I wanted to cast her. Same thing with Ginny.

But Missy is a Taurus in every sense of the word. She never makes a snap decision. She weighs her options. Sometimes, she waits too long but, then, my problem is the opposite of that.

For this film, we had auditions in January in 2019, and then again then in March, when Megan Jones and Virginia Beld travelled up from Knoxville.

All our second round auditions were there, too. Molly, Danielle, Katie (who was forty-five minutes late; it cost her the part of Missy. At fifteen minutes early, you're on time. On time, you're late. Fifteen minutes late, and you're fired.) She ended up with a small role that really didn't allow her to do much. But she was at the set on time, and she executed it extremely well.

Megan and Ginny came in, and we hit off, right off the bat. I thought that I really wanted to work with those girls, I'd hoped that Missy did, too.

The girls had oodles of natural chemistry. Thomas, they're best friends, and they a lot in common with you, more than you know. Megan struggles with depression, and a poor self-image. She lacks confidence, which is ironic because she's a little powerhouse actress.

Thomas called her Knoxville's best kept secret, but that was before she blew us all away with her performance in *Letters to Daniel*! She has the look, the chops, and she isn't a diva. She is without ego.

She doesn't say that I can't do such and such, or that I only have so much juice left. Ginny showed flashes of diva like behavior, but it wasn't like I thought, *Oh, my God, I can never work with her again*. She's an excellent actress. Even though she was a bit much sometimes, it was really nothing.

I have worked with total drama queens, bitches, and set divas. Ginny was nowhere on that level. In fact, it was just a matter of rolling the camera, and she would give it her all. Other women whom I have worked with tested me to my limits.

What I found when working with Megan was that she remained in character until I said, "Cut." Then, she went back to herself. Megan can turn on and off like a light switch. The one time I watched her go deep and have to decompress after a scene was the panic attack scene in the theater.

She did a helluva job portraying what it is like to be stuck in that mode and not know which end was up.

I think the hardest scene on Ginny was the funeral scene. With the noise of the thirty or so children screaming and kicking in the nursery, her concentration was really tested. She put herself in the headspace that it was her grandmother's funeral and that she was saying goodbye to her all over again.

Megan is a strong actress. She and Ginny continually hit it out of the park on each take. We often got coverage, but some people disapprove of my directing choices. It's not a slam on them, we simply have different styles of directing. I choose not to brutalize my actors by asking for double digit takes.

That's not to say that it doesn't work for others. Thomas has a way of winning his actor's trust that allows him to do that. It's not right, or wrong; it's just a different way to do things.

And, like I said, Thomas is freaking brilliant.

Me, on the other hand, I'm steadily learning how to take feedback and put it toward the next project. I choose to have a more relaxed hand and allow actors the opportunity to risk something of themselves; that's how I gain an actor's trust.

While on set, everyone pretty much behaved as they should. Without ego, people gave me their best. But every set almost always has at least one bad apple, and we had a creeper on set, whom I will never work with ever again. Stalking a married woman is just uncool and unacceptable. I'm embarrassed that it happened on my watch.

Thank God, she felt comfortable going to Mark for help, and he alerted me and Missy to the problem. Unfortunately, it was after the fact, and I wasn't cued in until the last shot of the shoot.

Be that as it may, one bad apple out of close to forty actors isn't a bad ratio. (That son of a bitch was married, too!)

Set life can be wonderful, such as the coffee shop. The aroma of coffee, and pastries, was just as relaxing as anything else I could think of.

The fourth and fifth days were the hardest. We had twenty pages and eighteen pages to shoot respectively. Doug did magnificently in pre-production. Without his organization filming, it would have been a disaster.

Even though his finger snapping drove Clint crazy in the editing suite, Doug was a great asset to mine and Missy's film. He fell in love with Ginny and Megan as performers and even took them out to breakfast on their last morning in town.

Megan and Ginny arrived at the audition before anyone else. Megan was good, and the only person whom I wanted. Another actress showed a lot of promise, but I needed the likability factor because the role of Amy would do highly unlikable things to Missy, but the audience would need to know it was because Amy was sick, not crazy.

While her audition hinted at things to come, it did not prepare me for how much of a powerhouse she really was. Some people (like William Goldman) say that they don't vote for physical, or mentally, ill characters when it comes to awards season.

But, here's the reality, portraying someone with a mental illness requires a certain balance. Some people want extreme emotion, and that does not always play well cinematically. But it's still their preference as a director, and their right. There's an audience out there for it, so who am I to criticize them?

Missy and I like our acting a bit more subtle. Our direction was, "You're sick, not crazy." There's a stereotype about mentally ill people: that we're all angry, isolated, white supremacists, and that is not what makes one mentally ill.

Mentally ill people are like anyone else, only we need medicine, therapy, and a lot of love because people assume an act of hatred is an act of illness. While aggressive behavior is a symptom, we are not prone to acts of mass violence.

Our acts of violence are of a more intimate nature, such as a fight I once had with my sister—not an argument, a fight. She got worked up, she got self-righteous, and she started attacking me verbally.

Usually, I let something like that go because it's not worth engaging her. But, for some reason, I'd had enough of her bullshit. As George Clooney says, "This shit over here, I'll eat. This shit, I won't eat." And, admittedly, my fuse had already been lit with people laughing at me, and dad getting worked up about me wondering why I hadn't been called to dinner. So, when she started ranting at me, I gave in to MY anger and did the smallest violin in the world playing with my finger and thumb.

Then, she punched me and proceeded to yell at me.

I know that I can take responsibility for my part in the fight, but I doubt that she'll take responsibility for hers. Everything is always someone else's fault. Even though she punched me, and I got up to punch her, neither one of us was going to get our hands on an AK-47 and annihilate innocent people because out temporary feeling of rage toward each other was misconstrued as hatred in our hearts for humanity.

And it was crucial that Megan be able to dance that line and create empathy for my character. Just as importantly, Ginny needed to be able to show, though frustrated with Amy at times, that she loved her like a sister who was, indeed, worthy of her unconditional love.

19

MY FIRST CHAMPION: PSYCHOLOGICAL SIBLING, L. ANDREW COOPER

I met Andrew through a publishing house that we both called home to our books, his *Burning the Middle Ground*, and my *Gemini Rising Series*. We first sat on a panel together at Conglomeration in 2012 with a mutual friend, Pamela Turner. We talked about portrayal of conspiracies in fiction. We also talked extensively about the *X-Files*, and butted heads. I thought that guy had a Harvard education, and considered himself better than me (which was not the truth of the matter).

I would try engaging him in conversation at various events, and we never connected. He seemed standoffish, so I assumed that he didn't like me. But, when I made *Letters to Daniel: Breakdown to Bestseller* and released the first volume in 2013 and 2014, he bought the book. He said that he had gone back and re-read his favorite passages.

In 2014, I entered Imaginarium's quaint little film festival with it, but not before entering Indie Gathering (where I would go on to win honorable mention). But, at Imaginarium, Andrew was a film judge. I didn't know if I would win. There was another documentary there, so the chances that I would win an award were good.

But Imaginarium is a three-day event where there are tons of panels and workshops about writing. The first year was a blissful experience. I managed to sell thirty books and take home an honorable mention. I was so tired and fried on the last day that I was angry. The other filmmakers didn't stay for the awards ceremony.

It was the bipolar disorder. I've learned to pace myself better since then. That, or I've grown stronger. I prefer to think that I've grown stronger. People who don't understand what I'm working toward, or see me as sitting on the computer all day and nothing else, don't appreciate how hard I work.

I put in crazy hours, and I will protect my creative ventures with my life. The creative ventures keep me balanced, and they keep me alive. When I'm not creating, it is a miserable existence.

Sara, my next to youngest sister, is thirty-nine years old. She busts her ass to give her boys the things that they need (with a lot of help from Mom, Dad, and the rest of the family). She works full-time and feels unappreciated in all aspects of her life. And, as a result, she is volatile emotionally; it's like navigating a minefield.

I could tell her what works for me, but she won't do it. And part of the Bipolar Clash of the Titans happened because she couldn't, or wouldn't, acknowledge her part in her recovery and illness. She'd felt put upon at work (Quite honestly, I wouldn't want to work with her, she's a total bitch to anyone whom she feels isn't as smart, or as good, as her) and was telling me how she wasn't irresponsible with her money. Ehh, wrong answer. She spent $500.00 on an ugly ass tattoo in remembrance of a guy who wasn't good enough for her, when she needed it for vacation just a few weeks later.

She accused a girl of never taking responsibility for her actions at work, and all I could think was, *Pot, meet kettle.* When I tried to suggest that she might want to probe her pdoc a little more about her diagnosis, she started yelling.

I usually walk away at this point, put I had hit my limit, so I started playing my heart plays for you on the tiniest violin in the world. She punched me, which triggered the hell out of me, then all hell broke loose, as I mentioned in the previous chapter.

It was bound to happen; she has absolutely zero respect for what I do, or how hard I work. While I'm not proud of what happened, I have apologized for my part in the incident. (I could have called the cops if I'd had my own place.) But, to be fair, cops are the worst at handling situations like that. Someone gets shot, or taken to jail, when what they need is a hospital and pdoc and therapist.

Making the proof of concept documentary in *Letters to Daniel: Breakdown to Bestseller*, I was attempting to tell my story so that I would heal and that others might know they could find healing and be in recovery.

What I couldn't possibly know was that the judge, Andrew, also had bipolar disorder. And, I when I won runner up, I was not in the headspace to be happy about it. In fact, I resented it. But it was 6:00 p.m. on the third day of the convention, and I wasn't feeling rational.

But I'm nothing if not a good sport, I plastered a smile on my face and accepted the trophy for runner up.

I wanted out of there. My tired and ill-equipped mind wanted to run as far away as fast as I could. The no talk rule was put in place, and it was a sad, silent drive home.

When I got home, I took my meds, fell into bed, and got a

good night's sleep. After a week of recovery time, I found that I had a fresh perspective. It was an award. I could put it on my bio. It marked the second time I received an award for a film I directed and that Missy produced.

It was a collection of twelve or thirteen letters with a collection of photographs of me from childhood to present. I did the voice over because I didn't know anyone who did that sort of thing.

It had a closing credits song, a beautiful song by Danny Jones called "The Wind Blows Through My Garden." He wanted me to use it in the narrative song, but Valyo's intro was more appropriate, and it sets the mood beautifully.

So I promised Danny that I would use the song, at least, in part, for my *Recovery Unplugged* show. It made for a beautiful opening.

But, as I said, Andrew was a judge, and he had fought for my film to get an award, so I approached him afterwards for insights as to what I could do to become a better filmmaker.

We talked over Facebook. And he told me the writing (the letters) was magnificent. But, of course, I had zero production value. It was then when I asked Missy if it was okay to send him *Letters to Daniel*, our narrative script based on the international bestselling memoir, and documentary, of the same name.

With much trepidation, she agreed. And I gotta admit that I was terrified. Andrew isn't cruel, but he doesn't sugarcoat his notes, either. If he doesn't like something, then he will tell you in a witty, and wickedly funny way. I told him I understand that he wouldn't sugarcoat, but to please be gentle; I was literally placing my life in his hands.

I waited a week and then messaged him. His verdict, he said he didn't know what to expect when reading my script, but he said that he needed to tell me something first. He informed me that he also had bipolar disorder, only his was bipolar 2.

This is something that happens to people who have seen the documentary, read the script, or any other iteration of *Letters to Daniel*. It becomes a gateway for discussions to be had, for people to bond, to share things that they have felt ashamed of sharing, and to finally feel like they're not alone. Others need to feel accepted for who they are and not worry about a judgmental voice on the other end.

They're home, in a way. And, when they're home, I'm home.

Andrew was home. He said, "Okay, let's talk about the script." He said he loved *Letters* and agreed that some of them were brilliant and amazing, but wondered how they would play when the scenes were going on. He also wondered how it would affect the film as a whole. Andrew also said that the first thing a Hollywood producer would probably do would be to hand it back to me and say, "Re-write this without the letters."

But he felt it was a very good script, and that I was extremely talented. Well, me and Missy were. I tend to say "I" a lot when, in reality, it's "we." Without Missy, the magic doesn't happen. She is the other half of my brain.

We managed to live together for twelve years and not kill each other. We came close a couple times but when you live through the fire of bipolar disorder, if it doesn't break you, it gives you a kind of superpower.

As a caregiver, as well as a consumer; that's the term for patient that is supposed to mean less stigmatizing. I'm a consumer. Andrew's a consumer. My cousin, Rebekah, is a consumer. My cousin, Logan, is a consumer.

All of us are in various stages of recovery. We've all had victories and setbacks over the years. My superpower is knowing how to ride the creative waves when they come. I try to always be in my creative mode. Some people marvel at my creative output. Some resent it. Others see me as a marketer, and little else.

Having set out to film a movie, and a feature film at that, I'm at that point where the only opinions I care about are mine, Missy's, our various mentors, and the audience *Letters to Daniel* is intended for.

I called Andrew my champion at the beginning of this. That's for many reasons. He loves the *Letters to Daniel* brand and what it has meant to my healing, and recovery, as well as other caregivers and consumers. He loved it so much that, for my fortieth birthday, he and his husband, James, drove me and Pam Turner to Nashville for Film-Com, where my project had been accepted to pitch to executives. I shared my table with Andrew and Pam.

Andrew and James paid for my hotel, a very swank hotel, for four nights. It was a luxury hotel, and they gave us a suite. Andrew promptly pitched *Letters to Daniel* as hard, as I was, and taught me a thing or two. Andrew is my best guy friend. I hope to see him next year at AOF Megafest, and I hope to give him a good return on his investment.

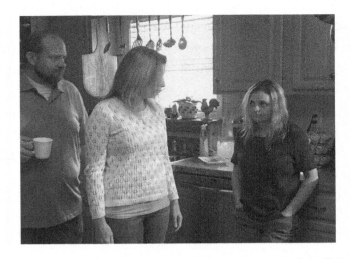

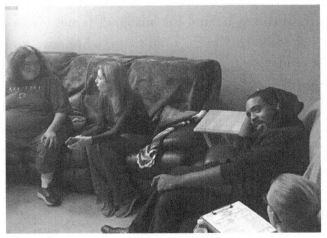

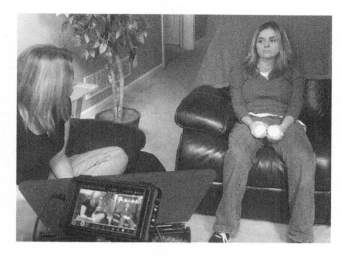

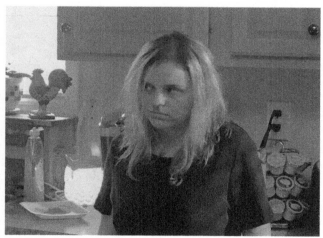

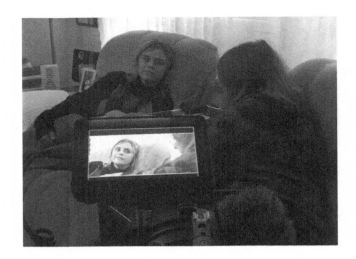

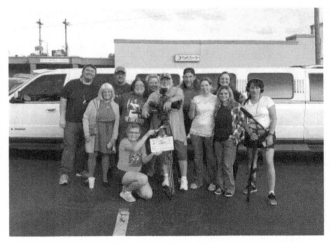

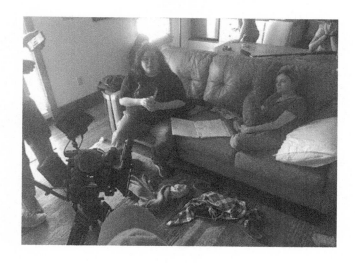

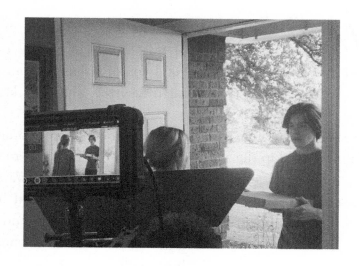

20

TAKE ONE, SCENE ONE, DAY ONE

e should probably start with the night before when people first started arriving. First lesson learned, drive to the motel or hotel you are housing your cast and crew and vet it. Don't end up with a clusterfuck, like I did.

I've already written about the terrible conditions. Bugs on the pillows, mold in the shower, having to pay for clean towels, having to replace your own toilet paper. Drugs, drug paraphernalia on the property. My script supervisor was asked if he wanted any ice. Then, we were ripped off at night, and our script supervisor was threatened with violence. The manager told us that he was going to call the police on him and threatened to physically throw him out.

The name and location of this infamous motel, the Intown Suites, 7121 Preston Hwy, Louisville, KY 40219.

Did I mention I love my cast and crew? They came from all over to be in mine and Missy's film. Oklahoma, Arkansas, Michigan, Tennessee, Ohio, a few from Kentucky. They had every reason to abandon me, and *Letters to Daniel*, upon sight of that motel room, but they stayed.

Mark told me, "Amy, if it had been anyone else, I would have taken my truck, turned it around, and gone straight back to Arkansas."

I housed a few of the ladies for a couple of nights while my mom and dad weren't home. Anna-Maria returned to the motel on the third night, and Abigail begged to stay. My mom acquiesced. God bless Mom and Dad. They often don't understand that I'm just as sick as my sister, but they do everything they can to support me otherwise.

I arrived on set on day one to learn I'd given everyone the wrong address because Google gave the wrong address. So I scrambled to give those who were lost the correct address. (Thank God for Facebook Messenger, and the fact it happened to be working that morning.)

Everyone pretty much arrived there on time, more or less, except for Marjie. She said that I could use her office. Unfortunately, there were about fifteen people loitering outside her counseling center, waiting to get in.

As I blew up her FB phone number for forty minutes, I began to sweat. Starting off from behind the eight ball wasn't exactly ideal. We were losing valuable minutes, and we had to be at the church by four to film a scene, and we were out by six. It was the week of vacation Bible school, and the recital was that day, Friday.

Finally, she answered. She was surprised to hear from me and said, "Weren't you supposed to be there Saturday?"

"No," I replied. "Today, Friday."

To her credit, she threw her clothes on, came up there and let us in before leaving the office and giving us the run of the place.

It took her twenty minutes to get up there, which put us an hour behind. But, thanks to Mark, we had gotten the exterior shots done. We took one more of Megan walking down the street to the inside. Julie Westlake Sooter slated, everyone else stood on the sidewalk, and I sat in a chair Mark provided me. Mark is one of my many heroes on this set. Because of his talent, and professionalism, we were able to move fast and get what I wanted at the same time

Because of his unique combination of teaching, and collaborating skills, I was able to communicate more effectively with my crew and become a better director. I still have a lot to learn, but you only learn by experience, so I'm gearing up for a documentary about my dad and me and how we have been running, or walking, together since I was twelve years old.

I started back at the gym last night, and I hope to keep it rolling, training for the Kentucky Derby Half-Marathon. That's 13.1 miles. It will be my seventh. While touring with *Letters to Daniel*, I'll have to train and utilize the hotel fitness centers (if they have one) along the way.

But day one was filled revelatory performances from Megan Jones, and just about everyone else, except for one scene. That scene was so even that, as we were filming it, I knew that it would be cut. There was really no saving it. Two of the actresses didn't know their lines, and they wouldn't speak loud enough for the boom mic.

Megan gave it her all but, as Clint said, it was the easiest cut to make; he dropped it like a hot potato. It pissed me off that the actresses couldn't be bothered to memorize their fucking lines. That was an important scene.

The other two pdoc scenes made the cut: the one where I am tossed aside and not taken seriously, and the scene with Megan's and Vanessa's and Julie's performances, which chilled me to the bone and took me right back to that night when I so desperate for help.

Justin, Missy's cousin, who was working sound, asked me, several times, if I was all right. It wasn't hard because it was behind me. It bothers me to think the one pdoc is still working and treating consumers.

My experience, while traumatic at the time, probably wasn't unique. Emergency room pdoc's are a dime a dozen. And, chances are, they're just as messed up as you are. A lot people like me (meaning those with mental illnesses) go into the profession because they want to help people. Others go into for the money. I've encountered great pdocs, and therapists—therapists with a good heart, but not much compassion for poor individuals who find it difficult to pay.

I've been fortunate to have consistent treatment. The second pdoc scene we filmed was fantastic. Ryan Yates had a nice, gentle compassion; he was able to tap into as our heroine finally puts a name to what has been tormenting her.

Megan did such a good job with the body language. I had been at the end of my rope during that time part of my life.

I had no place to turn to for relief. I was physically, mentally, and emotionally at the brink, and the only thing keeping me from going over the edge was Missy hanging onto me. And, even then, I was dragging her along for an unwanted ride.

After we wrapped on the location, Missy and I straightened up, packed the food and drinks up, locked up the counseling center, and everyone headed to Messiah Trinity Church to shoot a pivotal scene (which did not make the cut). It was the scene where Myra Hutton and her lackey, Natalie, stigmatized me then illegally fired me for having bipolar disorder.

It was a scene with a lot of voice over. Clint said it wasn't well-acted. I wish I would have put my foot down and had him add it back in, along with three other scenes. It would have given us the seventy minutes that we needed. But I pay him for his experience and, while I fought for five scenes, those others might have had technical deficiencies. Clint said that they cause a drag in the pacing.

Collaborating isn't always easy, but it is with Clint. I'm always learning, and he makes me feel like an equal, like he respects what I'm doing and why I'm doing it.

Not everyone does. Sometimes, I let the haters get to me. Those are the people who tear me down, the people who would like to see fail. But, after I got done feeling sorry for myself, I turned it into fuel to power when I feel like giving up on my dreams.

At the church, we dealt with unbearable heat. Sweat was pouring off of me, and Mark's shirt was soaked clear down to his waist.

Even though we did not use the scene in the film, I want to take the opportunity here to thank the talented Wynter Morris, and Madison Liesch, for driving all the way from Cincinnati on their own dime for one scene.

Timing was everything. When I got to the church, a member of came up to me and said, "What's going on here?" Dealing with difficult, and nosy, people is part and parcel to the. I didn't have fifty, or one hundred dollars, just to make her shut up, so I had to explain that I was filming a movie about my struggles with bipolar disorder and that I had permission from Pat Case, and Suzanne, to be there.

She gave me a little more bitchiness before laying off me then heading back into the reception hall.

That being said, the Messiah Trinity Episcopal/Lutheran Church has been nothing but supportive of me in my journey to make *Letters to Daniel* a reality. They supported my trip to AOF Megafest this year. I can't wait to do a potluck/special screening at the church to thank them for their love and support in that journey.

The first day was long and, when we had a delicious dinner of taco salad, I thought that I would get some sleep. But, during an independent film shoot, the director never sleeps. You're always preparing for the next day or catching up on your emails or sending materials off to a film festival. That's me, especially during the summer.

Missy was on set, and amazing all day. I feel like I collaborated more with Mark than with Missy. And, when she tried to give me input, I just gave her dirty looks. Not fair. It was wrong. And I want to apologize to her now for my behavior.

She is the most amazing person and, for those who have already seen *Letters to Daniel,* it's no secret anymore. She worked her ass off on the set of the film. She was the set mom. She comforted at least three people that I know of: Doug, Tim, and me.

Day wrapped, and we were pulling out of the parking lot of Messiah Trinity at 5:56 p.m. I was absolutely wiped out, and I knew the next day would be that much harder because I had to work. So I would not have the amazing Missy to assist me, guide me, or give me input. I would be leaning heavily on Mark, and Abigail, and, depending on them to monitor my temperature mood wise.

Usually, I'm good at pacing myself but, when I'm on a set, I forget. I forget to drink. I forget to eat. We got everything we wanted to that first day, and we got out on time. That would not be the case for day two.

DAY 2: ADVENTURES IN BEING LOCKED OUT, AGAIN

*W*ho says that lightning doesn't strike twice? Day one, I had been late to the set. Not good when you're the one responsible for running it. That was Missy's fault. She insisted on sleeping. There's not much time for sleep during the shooting of an independent film, but we were only late that first day.

Day two, we (Abigail, Anna-Maria, and me) rolled into the parking lot of the Ramada Plaza Conference Center and Hotel. About that time, everyone else did, but so did the thick, black clouds of a severe thunderstorm. Locked out, yet again, this time by another forgetful, well-intentioned person. Thank God Stephen Zimmer and Holly Marie Phillipe had Kippie's phone number.

As everyone else huddled beneath the roof from the rain, I did several things. I got Mark breakfast and proceeded to get worked up. Until an hour later Kippie, when answered the phone and said, "I thought you weren't supposed to be there at twelve with the wedding."

"No, ma'am," I replied. "I'm the filmmaker with the movie due to shoot here at 7:00 a.m."

She fell all over herself with apologies and explained that it would be another hour before she arrived.

Great. Meanwhile, Mark was parked under the roof, where his equipment remained dry.

Everyone was there but Tom Morton. I had seen him skulking about at the hotel but, clearly, we were supposed to be at the conference center behind the hotel.

Maybe I should've called out to him. As it was, we used Tony Acree to fill in. The ultimate irony is that the scene got cut altogether because there was no actionable audio, per Clint.

I was disappointed because it pointed out why the girls were heading to Texas, but I love the cut of the film that ended up with the sound editor/composer.

Day two, Mark and everyone really hammered down, and we managed to make up some time. We filmed five scenes at the hotel.

The first one was with Tony and the girls. They're full grown women, but I call everyone a girl. Now, to be fair, in the hands of some, the word "girl" is loaded and fraught with conde-scension. But, for me, it's a term of endearment, and affection.

The scene we shot was between Missy, Amy, and Jim Vaughn. It was a real life snapshot of a longer experience. Jim was an experienced scriptwriter who sixty-nine years old at the time, (he's probably passed on by now) who had "reached that point in his career where he could pick and choose his projects."

He proceeded to tell us about his friend's boat, christened the FUJAMI. (Short for Fuck You, Judy, I Got Mine). How Wilford Brimley changed his lines and got a good response from the audience, and it managed to piss both him and Noble

Wittingham off. The line was about his best friends he ran around with as a teenager.

One of them sold brooms door to door, and sold one to a blind couple who invited him in to eat. And the kid ended up eating in the dark because the couple had no need for lights. He drank a lot while we were sitting there, straight gin with ice, and he smoked like a freight train.

And, at one point, he got very emotional talking about his passion project *Maple Park* about those friends. One night, when he wasn't with them, their car stalled on the train tracks at the wrong time, thus killing them all.

It was obvious from his body language, and his tone, that this still haunted him. He also gladly told us about his wife; he said he put a ring on it to let people know she was his.

I still remember Jim after all these years, and my initial impression was that he was a dirty old man before I even spoke to him. The server was a bitch and wouldn't let us drink our Snapple and soda from the kiosk. He didn't like her attitude and promptly bought us a couple of soft drinks from the bar.

We kept in touch while we were in Texas. In fact, he had been avoiding the departed super agent, Mickey Fryerburg, which was ironic because Missy and me desperately wanted to meet him at the time.

The involving Jim couldn't possibly include all that but I wanted you to know that, even though he got cut from the final version of the film, he left an indelible mark on me and Missy.

You see, *Maple Park* was his baby. He dreamed of seeing it on television. The Bloodworth-Thomas's of *Designing Women* fame had optioned it, and were always telling him to change it. At that time, he was saying that he wasn't going to make any more revisions.

We kept our eyes peeled for it but, as with a lot of optioned projects in Hollywood, it never got made.

I took the lesson to heart; be your own champion, make shit happen by hook, or by crook. If I had the money, and the means, I would make *Maple Park* in honor of Jim.

But, with mine and Missy's career, I feel like the needle was just starting to move, with people requesting our work in Hollywood. AOF Megafest, and Indie Gathering, have both been instrumental in our growth as writers and filmmakers.

I took four years of growth. I shopped my film, packaged it, and still got rejection from people who did not take me seriously; I was sick of waiting for "the right time." There is never the right time, or perfect time, to do something as outrageous as make a feature film with hardly any budget.

I've learned I can wait for someone to do something for me, or I can do it myself. Doing it myself is harder, but I can do it on my own timeline. God bless Aaron Allen for coming on as an executive producer. Between his connections, and ours, we were able to raise $2,100.00 and that was the difference between getting the film made and not getting the film made.

We were able to house and feed our actors and give them some gas money. Everyone received IMDb credits, and we all lived to tell the tale.

The second scene we filmed in the hotel is really the second half of an experience, so I might as well talk about them in conjunction with one another.

The fifth scene we filmed took place in Doug Kaufman's station wagon, aka, Buck the Big Brown Beast. It was hot and humid. The rain had stopped, the skies had cleared to some degree, and only two of the windows on the four door vehicle rolled down.

The girls were baking in the heat. In the movie, there was

an argument between Amy and Missy when Missy realizes that the car is not starting.

Amy suggests asking festival goers for jumper cables. Missy doesn't want to do that. Amy suggests calling for a tow truck. Missy doesn't want to do that, either.

Back to reality. At that point, I was hot, (we were in Austin, TX) and we were still looking at a two-hour commute home. I didn't feel like sitting there anymore, so I hiked back to the hotel, where I asked a snooty festival goer if she happened to have jumper cables. If you've seen the movie, then you know what her reaction was. And it was probably naïve of me to think that, at a top tier film festival, people would have them, but you have to ask in a situation like that.

When I asked to use the phone, the clerk directed to the pay phone. Fortunately, I had some change on me. Missy eventually came in and we apologized to each other and went to wait for the tow truck.

The three other scenes we filmed at the Ramada before moving on to film at my parent's house was at the beginning of the film, where I was screening of the proof of concept documentary, and what a big night that was for me at Imaginarium. It seems like such a long time ago, but it was really only five years.

Then we filmed the ending, people walking into the screening. It was nice; we had about sixteen people on set. And Mark did amazing things to make it look, and sound, like a packed house.

Wrapped up about 2:00 p.m. and headed toward my house. My parents generously stayed at a hotel so we could film. Not that Luke (my big booty Judy of a tabby) was happy about all those people and equipment crammed into such a small space in *his* house.

The great part was that, with Mark's equipment truck parked outside, and equipment setting out, and John (because was allergic to cats) sitting guard, my neighbors were inquisitive about what was going on.

It was nice to have Tori Johnson on set. She didn't have to be told to work; she just jumped right in and made Mark a happy camper.

We filmed at the house until 8:00 p.m. and had a very late dinner. I had things to do, like send files to festivals, and return acceptance letters. Some, I'm sure, fell through the cracks given that I was directing a movie. But the important ones got through. The next day, we would have three locations to make. And, boy oh boy, was it going to be close.

22

DAY 3: A MOVIE THEATRE, A HOUSE, AND THE CHURCH

*B*y third day, Missy was back on set after a brief one day where she had to work her sucky ass day job, which shall remain nameless so that she doesn't get any grief from her bosses. It was a relief to have her on set. Directing and producing is hard and, while I did my fair share of it in production and had a full day the second day of it, I was glad to have Missy on set.

What I feared would happen, because I had carried the load in pre-production, and had devised the shot list was that I would not be very open to her directing input. And it wouldn't be because I didn't like her ideas, or trust her storytelling instincts, both are very good. It would be because I, on some level, thought that this was my movie when, in fact, it was our movie.

The first location we had on the docket for the day was Village 8 Theaters. Yes, I know that's an *Avengers* poster in the background. Yes, I know that's an *MIB* International standee that she races past. I'm hoping that we can have it rotoscoped out at the distributor's expense. But the first shot we took was of

Amy on the phone with her biological father asking for money. I called the actor to get him on the phone, and he was AWOL. Fortunately, we had the beautiful Luke Collins step in.

We had him hide in the bathroom and use Ginny's phone. With the brilliant Mark giving me different options, I felt that I could concentrate on the different actors' performances, especially Megan and Ginny and Brandon.

The movie theater resonance rested heavily on Megan's shoulders, and the success of the film was in Maria's hands, as well as the three main actors.

The second scene explored what it was like to have an anxiety attack. Between Megan's performance, and Mark's camerawork, I got a very really depiction of what it is like to experience one.

Anxiety is like that unwanted parting gift that bipolar likes to give. Sometimes, you literally feel like you're going to die from it. We went for fishbowl angle of the shot. A distorted extreme close-up gives the viewer a claustrophobic sense of what it's like to be trapped in a mind, and body, that is assaulting you. And, inside that moment, you're helpless to do anything about it.

And, for the final scene, we chose the triangle approach and executed a wonderful scene between Megan, Ginny, and Brandon, one where Brandon's character shows compassion to Megan's Amy and offers his support to Ginny's Missy.

To say that working with those performers was a dream is an understatement. At that point, we moved on to my Aunt Debbie's and Uncle Frank's and Aunt Jan's house, where we would film two important scenes. One with Amy sleeping, and her Aunt Jan is explaining to her grandmother that she wasn't just being lazy.

Note: My eyes were closed, but I heard every word my

grandmother would utter. She would find me to be lazy, and never quite understand. My grandmother felt that, if I got saved, then I would be healed.

But I'll say it once more for those of you whose seats are in the back: You cannot pray your mental illness away. I tried to. And what I've come to understand is that no God would put a human being through that. And any idiot who believes that it's God's will for a human being to go through that deserves to be tested by their loved one, who is at the mercy of the capricious beast.

You can't go without medication and, if you are one of those who are resistant to medication, them my heart aches for you because I remember the time when my illness had me by the throat. It was a living hell for me, and all those around me.

As it if I don't know which said of the bipolar bed I'm going to get up on. Maybe I'll be energetic, and inspired. Maybe I'll wake up, unable to concentrate, and end up vegetating in a chair in front of the television. And there are still days when I can't get out of bed, and I pull the covers over my head.

The last scene we shot at my aunts and uncle's house was between Amy and her grandmother, and her grandmother saying that she shouldn't take her meds; all she needed was to be saved.

First of all, you should know that my grandmother didn't understand the danger of suggesting such a thing to someone with bipolar disorder. It didn't matter what she said because *I* knew that I needed the medication.

Second, you should know that I'm a Christian, but that there is a ton of stigma in the church. People are often told that it's not God's Will that they be healed. Another filmmaker at Indie Gathering also told me his wife was bipolar, as was his son. I pity them. To have someone say that the God Who loves you purposely struck you with an incurable disease is simply too cruel to contemplate.

Megan really nailed the weariness, the hurt, and the love I felt for my grandmother, even though she actively stigmatized me.

Having your grandmother call you lazy when the world is steadily piling it on is not cool; it hurts tremendously. I think all of us who are struggling with mental illness can be considered fragile at times. We are all fragile souls, but that doesn't mean that we're not empathetic, resilient, and ambitious.

When getting well during the early stages of my recovery, it was frustrating. I wanted to advocate for those like me, to write a book about it, to let people know that they weren't alone.

What I didn't realize was that I had a long road to walk, that I had to get my head on straight, and that I had to learn not to be so myopic and see things from other people's point of view.

When you're as sick as I was, seeing beyond your own pain is impossible. Bipolar disorder wrecks your mind, body, and soul. When I arrived back in Kentucky, it really wasn't by choice. I felt like a complete and utter failure. Once home, the mania wasn't so much the issue, as a six month long depression was.

It resulted in several trips to the emergency room, where my mom would have handed me over to be admitted. In retrospect, it might have helped, but Missy said that she could handle me. There's a lot to be said for such kindness.

Not everyone is cut out to be a caregiver. My parents love me, and they support me, but I don't feel their respect. But I guess, until I don't need their help anymore, that that won't change. They'll be at the screening of Letters to Daniel at Imaginarium and will be at the awards ceremonies at AOF Megafest.

I don't think that they understand all the work it takes to put together any film, but they support me, and they don't charge me rent. They let me use my EBT card as I see fit. And, for the film, it fed everyone.

When we finished at my Aunt Debbie's house, we had one more stop for that day, Messiah Trinity. We sent Abigail ahead to unlock the church and meet everyone.

As we cleaned up shop, and helped Mark load the equipment up, I was feeling good about the footage we had gotten. However, in route to the church, there was Missy text. She wrote, *"You're not going to like this."*

The message was from Abigail. Apparently, the Sudanese congregation was there and, more than that, there were a bunch of unruly, undisciplined, screaming kids running all over the place.

Now, I was supposed to have the church free and clear Sunday evening. When we got there, one member of the congregation herded the children (all thirty of them) into the nursery.

John stood on the other side.

We then tied the doors shut and proceeded to try and film the funeral sequence. One actor was a no call, no show, and no response. And, just when I thought that my actress was going to have a nervous breakdown, Brandon opens the sanctuary door and said, "Amy, there's tornado sirens going off."

I thought, *WTF?* What else was going to happen? Really, asking a question like that on the set of an indie film is a bit like tempting fate. We eventually got the scene, but it took seven takes, and you can still hear the screaming children in the background.

Megan and Ginny were magnificent in their performances. The three scenes we shot at the church were incredibly heavy. With Brandon coming in as a knight in shining armor was perfect. Patrick didn't actually do that. It was a bit of dramatic license on our part. Missy said that she wanted a boyfriend for her character, so I expanded and embellished a bit on Patrick's role during our lives down in Texas. While he was an angel, he wasn't a boyfriend. Too bad, Missy could have really used one to lean on.

To my relief, the tornado warning was canceled, and we found our replacement, Harold. We then called it a day and got ready for day four.

23

DAY 4: THE CEDAR GROVE AND MYSTI PARKER'S HOUSE, THE TEXAS APARTMENT

a week out from production, I hit yet another road block, an Air BnB location fell through after they got cold feet about a film cast and crew descending on their property. It was a Tuesday, and filming would start that Friday. My back was up against the wall.

I asked my cousins, Jackie and Bugsy, to help us out. After that, they started acting funny. I swear, people are so god damn weird. They just say, "No" and don't hem and haw. If you don't want to do something, then I need to know so that I can move on and ask someone else who will say, "Yes."

I knew it was a long shot, but I asked my biological father. He just laughed at me and said, "No." Yeah, I know, he's a douche. Always has been, always will be.

I was at a loss. I was already filming at my mom and dad's (John, not Jerry) house and my aunts and uncle's house. I took breath and took a chance, and then I called Mysti Parker.

I asked her, told her that we'd be out of the house by 8:00

p.m. and would give her fifty bucks for her troubles. She said, "Yes" without hesitating. God bless Mysti.

We couldn't have made the film without her home. And let me just say, it's a beautiful home: salt water tank with fishies in it, a gorgeous kitchen, which makes the opening credits, a spacious living room, where most of the filming was done. Even by the door was lovely.

She walked out with her family and trusted us to take care of her home. The only thing we left behind was a sock.

But, that being said, we had twenty pages to film.

First shot was of the kitchen and it included John Spalding as Harold and Laura Masi Cline as Neshea. They were wonderful as were Ginny and Megan. Unfortunately, the scene was cut, probably for continuity, but it was still a shame to lose it.

From there, we move to the doorway. The scene was between Patrick and Missy. When getting the shots of Brandon, it was pretty simple. Natural light was used, and both Mark and Jules Leskiv, (our second sound person) and the slate, (whoever picked it up at that point) were able fit comfortable to do our jobs.

When it came to film, Ginny we still used natural light, but it was like a small circus coming to town on that small porch fitting, slate, me, Mark, Jules, and Brandon. Thank God that Ginny knew her lines, and both Brandon and she executed them well, so that we weren't out in the rain forever. The important thing is we kept all equipment dry and were able not to fall off the porch.

The beautiful thing about filming at Mysti's house was that it was so spacious and allowed us to set up the shot with enough room for the equipment, and the actors, with no problem.

It might have been a little close for comfort in the kitchen.

But that's because there were four actors in the scene a multiple crew. It was a tight squeeze, but we got it done.

One of my favorite scenes couldn't be used because the sound was only recording before the shot and after the shot. It was pivotal, and I lament it not being included, because Megan and Ginny were both so smashing in it.

Megan as me on the verge of losing control, and Ginny as Missy hanging onto me for all that it was worth. But things like that happen with indie films. Not cool, but we had another scene where you see the threads of my sanity unspooling, so there you have it.

Reviews from the gentlemen are always harsher. I know that they were giving me the benefit of their experience, but what I was really looking for was a, "You did good."

All the women who are psychological siblings of mine, Rebekah, Amy Wade, and Valerie were all moved to tears, and loved it. But, when you have the disease, it's easy to relate to my character. But all of them admitted to being mad at me for treating Missy poorly.

One thing the guys (directors, producers, and writers) were in agreement on was they felt that it was very brave for me to show how nasty bipolar disorder is (and I showed this in how I treated Missy less than what she deserved) and really being honest about the toll the disease takes on a household when there's not a lot people to help.

There was one scene where Brandon, Ginny, and Megan sit on the floor for a last meal together, and it cracked me up. Brandon, as always, is a dream to work with. The scene called for Ginny and Brandon to kiss. When I called cut, Ginny said to Brandon, "Man, your lips are soft."

To which Brandon replied, "It's that Cleveland water."

We ended the day on the pizza delivery for Christmas

scene, where Megan hands Michael (Laura's son) $12.56 in change.

To which he says, "um, um," and Megan just shuts the door in his face.

Watching it on playback and seeing the look on Megan's face cracked me, and the whole cast and crew, up. It was a great way to end the day on a light note. Then, everyone packed up and put Mysti's house back to the way it was, and we called it a day.

My feet never hurt so bad in my life. They ached in a way that made me wish, on several occasions, that I could just chop them off.

Missy drove us that day, so I didn't have to concentrate on knowing where I was going.

Now, I'm going back track a little bit. We started out at the Cedar Grove Coffee House in Shepherdsville, Kentucky. We enjoyed great toasted coconut iced mochas. The entire cast and crew showered business upon this locally owned establishment that welcomed us to use them as a filming location.

The setting was charming and, seeing that we were simply shooting two scenes, we figured that it would be a snap. Jules was on sound, and Mark was working his lighting genius. All the women got together helped John and Mark unload needed equipment, that is, those who were not focusing on the scenes. Ginny was in both scenes, so loading and unloading a truck wasn't something that she could focus on. Megan was essentially the star, as the film is told through her character's eyes. And, Anita. Well, she was old enough to be my grandmother, and she was playing my Aunt Rosie. She had no business doing anything other than acting.

We decided to shoot the girls (Megan and Ginny) with

Anita first. They had a nice relaxed chemistry. And, given the excitement of the morning, that was a good thing.

At the end of shooting on day three, the camera was overheating. So we worked blindly, without playback. Now, I've worked like that in the past, but *Letters to Daniel* marked new territory for me. The unease with this palpable for me and Mark, Missy may have felt it but, because I was living on the edge collapse, she was forced to bear my fear, and hers, inside her head. I dissolved into tears, fearing the worst, that we hadn't gotten those oh so important scenes that were crucial to the movie to show Missy's burden, and her humanity, how she was so much stronger than a lot of people give her credit for.

Ginny shed tears in the scene, and Megan looked so lost. It was an incredible performance on both their parts and, if we didn't have it, we would have been screwed. We had no way of filming at the church again, and we didn't have the time to do it over.

When Mark expressed his worry, and insecurity, over those scenes, my tenuous grasp on my emotions slipped and, for about twenty minutes, I descended into the ninth circle of hell. Fortunately, Doug, shortly before filming was to begin, made the announcement that the shots were indeed there.

The scene of Missy going to Patrick at the church was beautiful. Missy wanted more from Ginny but, taken in the context of the movie, she did a great job and Brandon, oof, he's probably the most generous actor I've ever encountered. To be fair, Ginny and Megan gave me their all as well.

This is an emotionally taxing tale for the audience, but the actors are drawing upon their reserves to really go for the emotional gusto that film called for without tripping into the "I AM ACTING" territory. The three main people in *Letters to Daniel*, you can't even see the seams of their acting.

That's when it gets really exciting.

The scene between Aunt Rosie and the girls went smoothly. They hit their marks, knew all their lines and we were onto the next.

This scene was between Patrick and Missy was to provide a counterpoint to Amy and Missy. Whereas Missy is always there for Amy, we took dramatic license and had Patrick be there for Missy.

What makes Brandon so good is that he makes the other actors around him better. Ginny is a solid actress, but she leveled up every time she was in a scene opposite Brandon. It's especially noticeable when it's cut together with the rest of the movie.

Ginny is a great actress. Her and Brandon together, well, it just gives me chills watching them.

The funniest part of the first part of the day was when the owner of the coffee shop came in and was blown away by the setup. He expected, maybe, a small camera, and a boom, but Mark is amazing with the lighting that he does.

I told him that I wanted the look of *Steel Magnolias*, and *Beaches*. In my push to put a dream team together, I stepped on Mark's toes a little bit during post, but I'll get to that later. On set, I felt like I had learned a massive amount from Mark, yet I felt like he took special care to respect that I was the director by always giving me options.

The truth was, more times than not, I deferred to his expertise, but it was always in line with the ultimate vision which I had for the film. Are there scenes we lost because of technical difficulty, or because poor acting choices? Yes, but that happens a lot on indie film. That's just the way of it. But some things that cost me are things I learned not to do the next time around.

I would work with Mark again in a heartbeat. I consider him a teacher, a mentor, and friend. He's an invaluable resource.

Day four required a side trip to mail off the first three days' worth of footage to Clint. Everything was raw footage and, somehow, he fashioned into something. When Valyo got through with it, it was very special.

The only hitch with day four was, when we went to shoot the exterior of Amy and Missy returning home. The dark clouds were moving in, but it was a very brief scene. I had secured use of the land next to a Five Star, but this bitch, queen god clerk of the world, said I didn't. I didn't know what I was going to do for a location for all the exterior shots. Tim would solve that problem at the end of the next day.

As it was, we got out of Mysti's house with ten minutes to spare, God bless, Mysti. Without her, and her family's generosity, we would have been screwed.

DAY 5: LONG DAY'S JOURNEY INTO NIGHT

*D*ay five didn't start until 3:00 p.m., so I got to sleep in and partake of Starbucks with Abigail at my parents' house. I slept until noon. The night before my feet had ached so badly that I begged my mother to rub them. God Bless her, she did. When Dad demanded that I move the car, I told him that I couldn't be bothered to move. We had filmed for thirteen hours the day before, so I was a bit belligerent, but I also knew that there was no use in defying him. In the end, it's my parents' car, and I can only use it some of the time.

Now, if my name was Sara Keough, I could wreck or damage every car they ever owned. Because, well, that's what she seems to do.

"Well, she has kids," my parents say when defending her. So, what am I, a single pringle chopped liver? I don't have a golden ticket. I know that my parents love me, I know that they support me, but I don't know how proud they actually are of me. Their eyes glaze over when I win awards now. With a total of 106 awards, most people are impressed. Mom and Dad just want me to do the dishes. But, truth be told, stuff like that keeps me grounded when I could very easily get a big head about it all.

Being gifted a film festival to execute a long held dream of helping artists with mental illness is a heady thing. I am the proud recipient of the Founder's Award at AOF Megafest.

I can feel my career about to explode. It really all rests on how well *Letters to Daniel* is received. Women love it; they are moved by it, and they get the context of the letters.

The guys are always very analytical, and they break down the material like a critic, and they tell me what they would have done it differently. I appreciate ALL the feedback I've been given. Even when I disagree with it, I make sure to thank them for watching my movie and taking the time to give me their thoughts.

Day five saw everyone dragging a bit. Mark's frayed nerves showed briefly, and that was when Missy and Abigail pulled me into the bathroom of the only location we would be at for the day. The two of them threw me for a loop.

They wanted to make the next day the last day of shooting and wrap in six days instead of eight. When someone with bipolar disorder is fixed on their routine, adapting isn't the easiest thing in the world, so it pissed me off royally.

Missy carefully, and methodically, laid out her argument out for this. I was so tired that I said, "Just do it, but *you* make the announcement." I was thoroughly rattled. But when Missy and Abigail made the announcement, everyone who had been dragging, or was cranky, rallied, and we had a brilliant day of filming.

The first scene we shot was the one of Amy and Missy seeing the apartment in Kentucky for the first time. I wasn't wild about the scene when we shot it, but it plays wonderfully in the film as a whole.

It was the excitement of a fresh start, being filled with hope for something better while still wrestling with the demons that brought us back to Kentucky.

I hate reflecting on Texas. A part of me still feels as if we failed, giving our enemies something to chew on and throw back in our faces. But, without our time in Texas, we wouldn't have *Letters to Daniel*. And, if I had to feel pain so that I would feel this bliss, then so be it.

The next scene we shot was a fight scene. Amy had been devastated by Children's World discrimination, stigmatization, and accusations that just weren't true. I felt, and still do, feel the sting of Missy staying on and getting a hero's sendoff, all it feels like to me is betrayal. All it feels like to her is lack of gratitude.

When filming the script called for Megan to spike the glass in her hand, she did it. We all jumped, and she broke character. The second time she did, it was perfect, and the cup broke into three different pieces.

That scene, I felt in my gut. All the old feelings of inadequacy bubbled to the surface, and the hurt and the anger I felt at Myra Hutton and her lackey, Natalie, was all too fresh again, and unresolved emotion about Missy remaining came back up.

It's hard to explain if you've never been stigmatized, or discriminated against, what it feels like to be pigeon-holed as a troublemaker for showing compassion to the more troubled kids.

It hurts. It demoralizes you. You feel guilt and shame. It's a lonely place to be. I wouldn't wish it on anyone. That may never heal. The fact they adored normal Missy and loathed weirdo Amy was a bitter pill to swallow.

They chose placating a father who was a little too friendly with the staff, and all the little girls, as opposed to having no time for the little boys. His daughter was hyper sexualized, and withdrawn. The signs that he was molesting here were there, at least enough to be looked at. Instead, they decided to fire me because he had money, power, and charisma and made them all feel like beauty queens.

I never trusted him. I did my duty as a childcare worker, and I got punished for it. I wish Missy would have walked out in solidarity with me. When you're treated like trash, you need your allies more than ever. I never felt so betrayed, and so alone, in all my life.

Missy reasoned that there were bills to pay, but I still think she should have walked out on them. She still believes that I need to see it from her point of view. It's one of those things we agree to disagree about.

The only exterior shot we got at the location that was doubling for the Kentucky apartment actually took place in Texas. The deck we shot on was gorgeous. The backyard was nicely landscaped. And Megan and Ginny were talking about Amy and Missy, and their initial move to Texas. Amy thought Missy understood that they would have to hit the ground running. Missy thought that they had two months to find a job. When, in reality, they had one month.

When we were in Texas, Missy freaked out at that point. Somehow, I talked her into to staying. If called upon to do what we did in Texas at twenty-four and twenty-five years of age at forty-four and forty-five both of us would be like, "Hell, no."

Surviving on spaghetti and hot dogs is not the life you want to lead. But it is exactly those kinds of sacrifices that have made us the people we are today, and it makes for a funny bit in the movie when there is a lot of serious shit that goes down.

One of the things I had the most fun doing was reliving that second Christmas. Getting to watch Megan and Ginny re-enact it was something out of a dream.

They had a natural chemistry and, compared to the

Christmas scene we shot the day before, this was all good vibes and warm fuzzy feelings. Ginny and Megan, along with Maria's voice over, really captured the feeling of that night, even though there's daylight flooding the room in the film.

The most telling scene we shot is when Missy sees that I made an international phone call that lasted forty minutes, and Missy flies off the handle. The reality is much different from Ginny's performance.

In reality, Missy totally lost her shit. I mean, it hit the fan in a very big way. She screamed, she cried, she berated, she threw stuff, and she slammed her fists into loveseat. She then went to her room and proceeded to shove everything off of her bed and onto the floor.

I carefully walked down the hallway and approached her. I was at the doorway and asked was it okay to come in. By then her anger at me, her grief over her dad's death, and rage at having everyone lean on her and depend on her, had been spent.

I had to rise up and be the kind of friend she deserved in the face of all that. Megan and Ginny did well in those scenes, but the reality of it was just so much more intense. But what works in real life doesn't always play great on film.

I believe that Megan and Ginny struck the right balance between emotion, and believability, without overacting.

The martini shot of the day was the aftermath scene, where I go to apologize to Missy, promise never to do it again, and comfort her. The sound is really bad right on that scene, hopefully Valyo can work his magic on it.

We were able to use the carriage house location because the people who owned it through Air BnB were generous and allowed us to do so. They were also extremely kind and helpful, and their home is so gorgeous that it made for a great setting.

As we shut down for the night and enjoyed some pizza, everyone pitched in to help Mark load up the equipment. At a loss for a location for the last day of filming, Missy called on the mayor.

Tim called Hippyhead of OG Auto and secured it for us with little trouble. He really saved my ass on that one.

As we headed out to our vehicles to head home, the owner of the carriage house saw us out and gave us a great review on Air BnB, so we returned the favor. Finally, we rolled out and hit the hay, the next was going to be rough.

25

DAY 6: HOT SUN, SUMMER IN THE CITY

*W*aking up on day six, the last day. It was our last day with the beautiful cast and crew I had been working with. It meant saying goodbye to all the hardworking folks who had helped my dream come true.

Anna-Maria would be flying back to Oklahoma. Megan and Ginny would be heading back to Knoxville. Mark, to Arkansas, Doug to Detroit, and Abigail to just outside of Nashville.

There were Kentucky bodies on set, too. Jules and her daughter, Viktoria, Tim, Missy's cousin, Justin, and me. We were excited, and charged up.

We all descended upon Hippyhead's OG Auto. Let me say this, Hippyhead rearranged his entire shop just so that we could easily film on his property. He acted in the film, but it didn't make the cut. He didn't ask for anything.

He moved cars, trucks, and tools to the back. He made a place for my actresses to change clothes. When he performed in the movie, he was wonderful. (Too bad he didn't make the cut.)

We filmed Amy and Missy's return home to Kentucky first.

God Bless Megan; she wore a coat in sweltering heat. God Bless both Megan and Ginny; the scenes shot in the station wagon were sweltering.

Well, Abigail, too; she shot a scene in Justin's car, and it was hot, ninety plus degree weather with high humidity. Initially, as Amy returns "home," Anna-Maria (who plays my mom in the film) is her soft place to land.

She does an exquisite job of finding what makes Mom so great.

I love my mom, but she is far from perfect. Although we get along more as adults, that's probably because, when I've been working, it's easier just not to talk. In fact, if I interrupt her sitcoms, she says, "Let's talk during commercials."

As if having a whole day of not talking is easy on me, it's not. I tend to vomit out words if I was quiet all day. This annoys Mom because she tells me and dad to shut up while we're out in the living room.

On set, though, it's organized chaos, to a degree. You have the shot list, but you almost always start with it only to deviate from it. Me and Mark were on the same page, so we got more coverage for *Letters* than I ever received for my other films.

On two separate occasions, Ginny was called upon to drive, and Doug absolutely freaked out. Understandable, Buck was and his only mode of transportation. If something had happened to his vehicle, he would have been screwed.

The first scene where Ginny drove, Mark, Abigail, and Jules piled into the back, and Mark totally stole the shot. Unfortunately, the shot did not make the cut, and it would have lent itself to the pressures we faced down in Texas.

Missy had been exhausted at that in the trip, and so had I. But I was cramped, and desperately needed to stretch out my legs. Missy didn't care; she thought I was doing it just to piss her off.

Now, I had to trust the filming to take place while I stayed seated. It was so damn hot. People were slamming back water and Powerade like it was going out of style. When they finally got back, Ginny was thoroughly excited to have driven "a woody wagon."

The next scene was Megan at Brakeway, on the phone with Ginny. Dylan Francis Calvi had his one scene in the film (besides acting as script supervisor). Unlike other scenes for which I had directed him, he didn't go over the top. He was very subtle, natural, a complete asset to getting mine and Missy's film done the way we wanted it done.

After that we took a lunch break, Missy said, "I've got to get you out of this heat." She was right.

I ordered a lot of food, but I could barely eat it any of it.

We tried to keep the break short.

Missy wasn't wild about carting other people around because there were times when she wanted to speak to me privately.

All I could think the whole time we were on break was, *Get back to the set, get back to the set, get back to the set.*

I was obsessed with getting all our shots before Hippyhead got tired of us, or just got tired of being at work.

One thing I will say, Hippyhead is the coolest location provider. He went out of his way to make sure that we had what we needed. When a woman who owned an adjacent business came outside and gave us the stink eye, I wondered if there'd be trouble. And, indeed, there was a wrinkle.

She called her landlord, and the prick came and said, "Who's in charge here?"

"I am," I replied.

He then demanded to see "Brian."

Tim said, "I don't even think Hippy's wife calls him Brian."

Hippy squashed his concerns.

Tim also remarked, "Anyone who refers to Hippyhead as Brian must be a prick."

Getting into the rhythm of filming after lunch didn't take much effort. The first scene we shot was another driving scene, where Amy and Missy are arguing. We needed another car, rather than Buck. We asked Justin if could use his car. What a sweetheart; he said, "Yes" without any qualms.

Granted, Doug wrestles with other demons, and losing control isn't his strong suit.

I was especially thrilled about having Justin on set. Whatever we needed him to do, he did, and he did it without complaint.

That day, he offered his car and assisted Mark with the camera after Anna-Maria's departure.

Another angel on set. Anna worked her ass off. Without her, I don't know what I would have done. When it came time for her to leave for the airport, we all got a little emotional. With the exception of the motel hell, the filming of the movie had been an absolutely beautiful experience, the most beautiful that I have ever had the privilege of being a part of.

Tim departed to take her to the airport. He said that didn't know if he would make the evening shoot because he had band practice.

I told him that he had better be back. But this was music. And, after the dissolution of his part in LAME, I knew the second chance meant the world to him. That doesn't mean that I wasn't irritated. I angrily assumed that he wouldn't show later on.

As we went on to film Megan and Pam in the car together, it

got to be 3:30 p.m. After we got the shots we needed, Hippy let us know that he wanted to close up shop. I was upset. We stood to lose another scene, the man on drugs scene. There was no time to film it, so we had to move it to later.

Missy dropped me and Abigail off at the house.

Abigail got a shower. (We sweated buckets basically from 8:00 a.m.-3:00 p.m.) Abigail was able to drift off. I had no such luck.

My parents fixed dinner that night. Then, Abigail and I headed to the Christy Cox and Associates doctor's office.

Everyone was so friendly, and kind. I had paid one hundred dollars for the location. That's just the price locally of getting things done. Corporate entities are impossible for small units, like myself, doing business. Yes, by definition I'm a production company but, usually, the general public thinks of studios. There is a studio in Louisville; it's located in the Portland neighborhood. But, then again, not everyone on the public thinks about.

My film's budget wouldn't even pay for people to have lunch on a studio film. The cast and crew I worked with were tremendously talented, hardworking, and dedicated. They did a lot for either peanuts, or no pay at all. I was blessed that those wonderful people did not turn on me and that Missy was there to do the things I could not.

As Mark pulled his truck and film trailer into the parking lot, we set up in the waiting room of the doctor's office. There was the scene with Rosie, Norma, me, and Missy driving the wrong way down a one-way street. We cut the scene, however, because I didn't feel comfortable having Mark's film truck there without John, or Brandon.

We shot the interior scene first. Megan looked like I did that night. We don't resemble each other, but the emotion she was

161

putting out there was incredible. She looked like she was on the verge of a nervous breakdown. It was a breathtaking performance, and I hope that it scores her interest from an agent (or agents) in Hollywood. I fully intend on giving a link to the former studio executive to look at.

The last scene we shot was "the man on drugs" scene. We needed an actor. Doug has a very distinctive look. We couldn't use him again, so we recruited Justin.

He came to the set fully prepared to work. He had a knit hat on. His face was smudged to look grimy, and he couldn't wait to be in it.

As we set up to film, I could feel a certain sadness, and satisfaction, setting in. I had labored for four years to get to that point. All the sleepless nights, all the tears, all the setbacks, and all missteps were finally worth it, as we were shooting the last scene.

When we called cut, it was time to call, "That's a wrap," to which Mark Maness treated us to a full rendition of "Rapper's Delight."

Afterwards, I hugged Mark, holding back tears, and I thanked him. He and Missy were my twin guiding lights. Now, it was time to transfer the footage and get it off to Clint. I had done it! I had proven all the naysayers and haters wrong, and I knew that we had a beautiful movie in the can. And, after my post-production team got a hold of it, I knew that it would be a beautiful thing.

26

DEALING WITH HATERS ON THE HOMEFRONT

*W*ell, to be fair I would call them doubters rather than haters. People really don't take me seriously as a filmmaker on the local scene. Maybe a little more so now that some have seen me in action with a cast and crew.

Or, maybe, they see me as a one note wonder. It's taken six years to build the beginning of a reputation as an advocate there. It's not that I'm completely hated locally, I definitely have my supporters.

It can be easy to give in to all your inner doubts when your critics make you feel like little more than a check to be cashed. I have to admit, the last couple of years at Imaginarium had left me with a sour taste in my mouth. It wasn't that I didn't love my Imaginarium peeps, it was just clear to me and Missy at least, that there was a pecking order, and we weren't on the list at all.

How do you make peace with spending a lot of money on Con, and every silver legacy since 2014 has received the sponsor award but Healing Hands Entertainment? And, every year, the definition of the award changes. Since 2016, I've come to terms with the fact we're never going to get it. There most definitely is a pecking order but, when I needed a projector for a scene in *Letters to Daniel*, Stephen Zimmer and Holly Marie Phillipe came through in a big way.

They got up at 4:30 a.m. and drove from Vevay, Indiana to the Louisville Ramada Inn on day two of filming. They didn't bring a sound system, so we were unable to use it. But, no matter, I needed Stephen to play himself, and he did. And, in a little revisionist history, Holly was at the first Imaginarium, too.

I was touched that they would travel all that way for me. Did I still feel like a check, maybe a little, but I was going into Imaginarium with so many good things that year. I launched three new books. I screened three webisodes of *Recovery Unplugged*. And I presented a workshop about thriving creatively while coping with serious mental illness. And of, course the test screening, and after party for *Letters to Daniel*.

You can laugh. The last few years at Imaginarium have been a big fat bust, except getting to spend time with my friends. I'll see Thomas this year because he won't be leaving for his internship until next year.

That being said, Imaginarium looks to be exponentially better this year. It would be nice to win an award there, but that hasn't happened since 2016. The judging panel definitely have their biases and preferences in material.

I don't foresee *RISE* winning anything. Although it is in the sci-fi/dystopian/fantasy vein, it is political, and my attempt to deal with the 2016 election, which profoundly affected me in negative way. The judges are pro-Trump, *RISE* is a distinctly anti-Trump manifesto. I'd like to think they wouldn't let that interfere with how they judged projects, but *Black Gold* called Trump out, and it cost me the screening. It's not an impunization of the judging process at Imaginarium. It's like anything;

know your audience. And what they like from me is mental health advocacy projects. That's the prism they view me through, for better or worse.

I also have a feature screenplay in competition, a drama about a man's coming to terms with his bisexuality. It's not sci-fi/horror/fantasy, so chances are that it won't win, either.

As for *Recovery Unplugged*, they might throw me a bone and give one of the webisodes a runner up. Fact is, while it's great content, Thomas's pilot, *The Devil's A Lie*, has better production value. Albeit, the fact that I would have directed it differently doesn't make it any less brilliant.

He desperately wants a best director award. I know the feeling. And when I won my first one at Low to No Film Fest this year, it was an incredible feeling. To be singled out for that award is something I'll always remember. What I desperately want is a best director award for *Letters to Daniel*.

Imaginarium has a quaint film festival. Do I question some of their programming and who and what they consider the "best," I suppose that I do. One thing I know for sure is that they do love film, and writing; their tastes just run a certain way.

Kylie Jude is one of the sweetest people I know, and Eric and Stephen are thick as thieves. I mean that in a good way. So, even if I don't always agree with their selections, I know that they sincerely think those choices are the cream of the crop.

I know they're starting to get really great scripts. Jeffrey Howe entered his *Coldest Horizon*. It's been winning everywhere it goes. Tony entered his *Hand of God* screenplay. Those scripts are fantastic, and they're written in a genre the judges at Imaginarium prefer, not that they wouldn't give it to a drama script. They just hadn't during their first three years of the unproduced screenplay competition.

I don't foresee them starting now, either, but that's not

necessarily a bad thing. Some festivals are comic cons, and that's what Imaginarium is growing into. It's not what I would want for my festival, but it's very clearly what Stephen wants. And, in 2019, there was considerable expansion in the area of multimedia talent, and not just writers.

Growth is good for Imaginarium, and I'm happy to see it. ISA (the International Screenwriters Association) recently came on board as a sponsor, and so has Spalding University's MFA Writing Program, two very big steps toward legitimizing their convention. That, and they were named the best writing convention in the region.

They seemed to be turning a corner that year, and I was very happy for Stephen. They went from a conversation with Lee Martindale at a disastrous for writers Fandom Fest, (although I always sold well there, despite my past with Ken and Myra), to what could be their best year yet.

So, while there is an element at Imaginarium that does not take me seriously as an artist, it is not just one festival director, or its judges. They might have a narrow view of what I can accomplish, but I'm hoping to change that when I test screen *Letters to Daniel* for them.

When the hate comes from the home front, it's a bit more difficult to deal with. Sara (my next to youngest sister) remains angry because she's not physically in the film, but she is mentioned in a very pivotal scene, he one where I go to the hospital desperate for help and am told it's all in my head. I mention that I have a sister with bipolar disorder, so it's not like I've erased her from my past.

I love my sisters, but my relationships with them are complicated by the past. They have reasons to hate me, and I have reasons to hate them. I love Mom, but she often pitted us against one another so that she could control our behavior. She didn't have to do much to control me. I was a good kid, never going anywhere that I shouldn't. I set my own curfew, and followed it. I got good grades and was an overachiever.

The rocky road started in my junior year. I suffered my first major depressive episode. As Mom and Dad applied the pressure for perfection, I internalized that it was like being in a pressure cooker. I got so depressed that I found myself standing at the kitchen sink a knife at my wrist.

Something pulled me back from the brink. I called my friend, Jason Denham, and told him how I was feeling. It was probably the most intimate talk we'd ever had, or ever would have. I'm pretty sure that I freaked him out. We weren't close, but I was feeling alienated from my girlfriends, who despised each other, probably because one slept with the other one's boyfriend.

Being suicidal is the worst. It's your own mind turning against you and flooding you with all kinds of lies, such as, *You're no good. Nobody loves you. Nobody likes you.* And, if your mind is especially cruel, and you have bipolar disorder, you could also start getting the everyone is against you thoughts when, in actuality, they are really rooting for you.

So the ultimate battle when dealing with haters is with yourself versus yourself. Are you going to give in to that part of yourself that exists in all artists? The insecure, sensitive part that allows you to create without abandon?

I don't think Imaginarium actively hates on me; they hold a special place in my heart. They were the first festival to actually screen my proof of concept documentary, *Letters to Daniel: Breakdown to Bestseller*. There was a lot of love in the room that night.

I wouldn't go so far as to say that my sister hates on me, she just demonstrates an utter lack of understanding where it comes to my career, what she perceives me as just sitting at the computer all day.

What I wish I could tell her, and that element at Imaginarium that thinks I'm not a serious artist, is that I work hard, I take calculated risks, and I seize opportunities when they're afforded to me. I hustle, I grind, but I also understand that publishing a book and distributing a film are the business side of the art coin.

I create to keep myself sane. But, in the end, I want to breakthrough to the mainstream, just like you do. Only, I have the ability to see the long view. This business is a marathon, not a sprint and, if I can be in recovery with bipolar disorder, then I can do anything. The real haters be damned.

ALICIA JUSTICE, FANDOM FEST, & DFWB

*E*very writer wants representation. It's one of those things that signals that you've made it to a certain level of professionalism. At the 2013 Fandom Fest, I met Alicia Justice. She owned JitterbugPR at the time and was looking to sign a bunch of clients. At that particular Fandom Fest, it was like shooting fish in a barrel.

She had been promised electricity so she could do her show and interview writers and, of course, the owners screwed her over. In retrospect, it takes one to know one.

I hired her to be my publicist but that quickly fizzled out, and she disappeared into the ether. A few years passed, but I kept in touch with her. In 2015, I entered the now defunct EPIC awards with my first volume of *Letters to Daniel*.

The first volume hit #2 on Amazon in the USA. And, when the judging for non-fiction was over, I was privileged enough to be a finalist. Armed with this, and a multitude of titles on Amazon and various other vendors, I approached Alicia to be my agent.

She thought about it and said, "Yes." She hung out her shingle, and I was her first willing victim—er—author client.

In the beginning, she showered me with attention, and we became friends. As the year progressed, I wrote a trilogy inspired by how outraged I was at my parents supporting a gentleman who had been busted for having child pornography on his computer, and disseminating it. They argued he didn't know that they weren't eighteen and, therefore, he wasn't guilty.

They also argued he didn't do anything to those girls and, therefore, didn't deserve such a harsh sentence. Knowing someone who was victimized this way, this infuriated, and sickened, me and led me to write an entire trilogy with villains inspired by the gentleman, and my parents.

I love my parents, but using your religion as shield for a criminal makes me sick, even if you are my parents. They visit him prison. I hate that. They judge Father Allen for cutting ties with him. For chrissakes, they don't see the crisis among priests being pedophiles, Father Allen can't be associated with someone who downloads and distributes child porn.

Anyway, Alicia told me that she had submitted to Simon and Schuster, and several other well-known imprints. I dutifully scribbled away. Writing three books in one year, and countless scripts of all lengths.

All the while going to my blog and discussing life with bipolar, and what I was grateful for. Gratitude and resentment cannot co-exist, so Magie Cook says. So, even though it chaps my hide that my parents try to justify his behavior and excuse him, I can choose not to engage them. I was so pissed at Dad that night that I punished him by only going to the gym for fifteen minutes. He hurt my feelings, so I shirked my training for the KDF mini-marathon. How smart was I?

I just choose happiness, and I do things that facilitate. I listen to music as I'm writing.

Alicia had a great poker face, and she hoodwinked a lot of people. She told me things like she had sent my book to Daniel Craig. That she had sent my script of *Letters to Daniel* to Sam Mendes. Of course, she said that the response was "no" to a foreword and "no" the directing the script.

As time passed, she became increasingly uncommunicative, unreachable, even on the simplest of things. She signed a lot of people because I encouraged them to. She wasn't moving anyone's books. The last straw for me was when she announced her own book deal after delivering empty promises to me, and several other authors whom she represented.

While that was going on, me and Missy were in pre-production for *Letters to Daniel*. That was all the way back in 2015 and, without therapy for nine months, I was barely hanging on to my sanity.

Then, nine days out from production, I received Facebook message at 2:00 a.m. from one of the other producers/cinematographers who was freaking out about their equipment and having the right cards.

I was not in a place to handle someone else's crazy, given that I was dealing with my own. I reached out to their producing partner. First on FB, then multiple times by phone, but I heard nothing but crickets.

I was faced with a devastating reality. I had a full cast, locations, but my crew was as flaky as hell. I could forge ahead with chaos sure to erupt on my set, or I could pull the plug, contact everyone, and regroup.

For the sake of my sanity, I pulled the plug. I was devastated. The first person I had to tell was Missy. Then, the casting director, who had so generously given her time and resources to help us procure a cast, was furious. She told me I had to make the movie, or my reputation would be ruined. Then, she proceeded to dump us.

I know that she had a business to run, but it just goes to prove that it's what you can do for people that interests them, it's another unwritten rule of show-business. So, when people come to me, I always wonder what their angle is.

I was devastated, and this served to destabilize me. I cried. After an initial rush of relief, severe depression set in. I bounced back and forth between mania and depression, which left me vulnerable to the people behind a local convention.

We sat for two hours of them telling me that I shouldn't be a writer, but a speaker. I would be free to create. Little did I know how, however, toxic their brand of "support" was. They manipulated me. They beat me down. By the end of my time with them, I was in a full-blown manic state, and suffering from PTSD from my time.

To be fair, I knew who these people were when I placed myself in their path, but I had gone from a liar to an abuser. The man liked to play head games with me and, honestly, he fancies himself a Svengali, and he thinks that he's way more intelligent than he actually is. She loves her husband. As people who didn't acknowledge mental illness as a thing, my time with them was destined to end sooner, rather than later. And their active attempts to separate me from Missy is ultimately what did them in.

I did what not a lot of people had done up to that point. I said "No" to them and left them. They threatened to come after me if I badmouthed them, but I was traumatized because of my time with them, and they say that, in order to heal, you have to share your truth.

The thing about people out to con you, you don't have to

take the low road. A year later, their comic-con went up in flames. All of their A card draws had cancelled, even Jim Cornet (a local wrestling star). He said that those people must have known something that he didn't.

When the next year came, they couldn't get enough vendors to commit. Their event didn't even happen at all last year.

It would be all too easy to do a little jig on that show's grave, but I do have gratitude for the early role that it played in my writing career. It's how I came into contact with Stephen Zimmer, and he is a stand-up guy with integrity. Do I always agree with him? No, but I know that he's not out to get one over on me.

That's why I continue to give my business to Imaginarium. I had high hopes for 2019, but not for the awards; I've let that go.

Letters to Daniel is test screening, I'm teaching a workshop, having an after party, am launching three books, and *Recovery Unplugged* is screening, the first three episodes to be exact.

The irony is I went from psychologically abusive situation to a chaotic one. Dragons, Fairy Wings & Butterflies signed me after I left that situation I mentioned above. I learned things that I didn't want to know about this person. What I'd learned by the end of my term with her was that she was a chronic liar, and an unwell woman. I don't feel any ill will toward this person, but drama = stress, and stress = anxiety, and anxiety = mania, or depression.

She lied about some very BIG things and, while forgiveness comes easy where she's concerned, it doesn't mean I have to break bread with her anytime soon, if ever.

So I left to her fold and like dominos, and other people who had signed with her left her as well. She blamed me. Maybe some of the others did leave because of me, but she had lied to them, too.

That being said, she taught me a lot about how to work on a film set, and what not to do. I feel like my first super successful film, *Black Gold*, was more her film than mine. But I'll admit that I learned a lot. And, without the experience on that film, I would have never have had the good fortune of eventually filming *Letters to Daniel*.

So the search for the manager/agent/lawyer team continues. Recently, an opportunity presented itself. We shall see where it goes.

MOM & DAD, THE SUPPORTERS WITH A LEARNING CURVE

*L*ike a lot of creative people, I have a love/hate relationship with my loving, but dysfunctional as hell, family. Some of them perceive me as being lazy and taking advantage of my parents.

You see, for thirteen years, Missy and I had not only worked together, but we also shared an apartment. First, in Texas, as shown in the movie, then in Kentucky. The amazing part about Missy about is that she stuck me through it all. And the reason why I put her at the top is not because my parents weren't supportive; they were and still are, but they were who I was assigned as a child by the universe. None we had a choice in the matter.

Missy did, and still does, have a choice. Sometimes when we argue, the gloves come off, and they used to come off all the time. Now, we're both in therapy and are more stable and grown up.

My parents, well, they are major supporters. Because now that I am an adult, they have no obligation to me. Do I hate some of their choices that they made when it comes to the company they keep? Yes, but I have to realize that it's none of my business. It only becomes my business when they want me to feel the same way.

Anywho, my mom has changed a lot from when I was in high school. The disease was ravaging me at the time, and we didn't even know it. But my mom said she noticed that my highs were very high, and my lows were very low.

But people weren't talking about bipolar disorder. Words like PTSD, and depression, were around but even those things weren't openly discussed.

They're saying that it's an epidemic now. I think it has always been an epidemic; people are just starting to speak their truth.

As I was saying, Mom first signed up as a caregiver when I got back from Texas in October of 2000. I had gone to a therapist when I was in high school, but she angry at my version of events. To be fair, the therapist didn't know what was wrong with me. Was my mom abusive to us kids growing up? I wouldn't go so far as to say that. Do I think she was suffering from mental illness in retrospect? Hell, yeah. She now takes an anti-depressant, and life with her is much easier. And it's easy to forgive some of her extreme behavior that I remember as kid because I know she was doing the best she could while coping with an unseen enemy.

Here's thing, as angry and alienated as I was at times, she always loved me, even when it got violent. Two intense, sick people clashing is a scary thing. It only happened once, but here's hoping that it never happens again.

During October of 2000, I was a shell of the person I used to be. Broken into a million little pieces, I returned to Kentucky, not by choice, not by design, but because I was so sick that I couldn't hold a job, or function in any real sense of the word. I wasn't even writing.

I was miserable. I felt that I had lost myself in the diagnosis. I couldn't separate myself from the disease. I was drowning. I hadn't gotten a full table of treatment. I'd only been prescribed medication. And, while medication is important, you need spiritual guidance, therapy, a healthy diet, exercise, a good night's rest. You also need an understanding, and resilient, support network.

Mom and Dad were at the gas station to pick me up for a few days, while Mom got me hooked up to services that I desperately needed. Gayle Sublet provided us with the number, and the names of some vocational rehab services, where I was evaluated and given eighteen therapy sessions, and eighteen psychiatry appointments. I wondered if they expected me to be "cured" of bipolar disorder that easily. It just doesn't work like that; I knew it. I was sicker than I'd ever been with the disease. It didn't make me stupid, but being without insurance made me a moving target for the government at that time.

I applied for disability, and they denied me. Shock. I let too much time pass but, with my Dad, and the mediators at the social security offices, and I appealed and reapplied. I was so broken at that time. There was so much paperwork involved, and I was just incapable of filling that stuff out.

Between Mom and Dad and Missy, I got all the paperwork taken care and, from there, was placed in a waiting zone. I didn't hear anything for months, so I figured that I wasn't going to receive disability.

During that time, I was stuck in a chronic state of depression. I would go over to my aunts and uncle's house, where my grandmother lived to and would sleep for hours on end because I just didn't have to the capacity to do anything else.

Sometimes, I would have my eyes closed but I would hear my grandmother saying things that hurt my feelings. They showed her ignorance about mental illness by forever assuming that I was lazy. When I just couldn't face the day, or handle being alone, I would ride along with Missy on her way to work (one of her jobs was that of a bus monitor for an elementary school where the kids adored herm and hated Ms. Sharon) where she would drop me off.

When the strong depressions hit, Missy had her limits. Then, I would go back to Mom and Dad's for a while, where Mom would comfort me, give me Chinese food, watch sitcoms with me, and basically just try to find a purpose.

Early on in my recovery my parents so the face of depression most of the time. The mania, or the rage really didn't show its hand to her. Most of the time it was Missy who saw the anger and different symptoms of mania.

Mom and Dad had to learn, I didn't want to hospitalized, because I never really reached that point. A crisis stabilization unit, on the other hand, I probably would have benefitted from. But, still, I had an almost irrational fear of having my rights stripped away from me. Missy inherently understood and would always vouch for me when my Mom and Dad, most likely, would have handed me over to the psych ward.

The reality is that the current administration is talking about the involuntary committal of all people with mental illness. That is a terrifying thought, one that drove me to pen a television series, *The Guardian*, and a novel covering the same ground featuring the same characters.

In 2011, I was starting to blossom. Creatively and professionally, I was starting to find my way by discovering the power of my voice and slowly beginning to turn a corner. I weighed

310 pounds. And, looking back at pictures of me then, I'm somewhat horrified.

My mother and father were concerned. In 2012, the pressures of living in poverty, and not being able to fully pursue my passions made me very aware that (go to more conventions, film festivals, signings) I needed a way to save money. I told Missy in January that, if we didn't stop fighting, I wanted to move back into our respective parents' households because I didn't want to start hating her because I couldn't grow as an artist.

In June, we made the decision to move back official.

Even though this was for the best choice I had made during that time, it was very hard for me. For the first twelve years of my recovery, I had lived with, and depended on Missy almost exclusively. I shunned help from my parents because they were always cutting me loose to help my Aunt Debbie, my sister, Sara, or Brandy. I neither needed, nor wanted, their help, so moving back was hard on me.

Dad said it more than once, "It's harder for you to live with us than for us to live with you." Very true. They didn't understand how powerless, and helpless, I was living under their rule. Early on, it was very bumpy. They resented Missy, though they wouldn't say it now. They caught glimpses of what Missy faced in the beginning since August 2012. Mania, mixed episodes, my sensitivity to sound and light. Glimpses but, unlike what Missy had endured, they got me fully equipped with my mental health tool belt.

They used to say, "St. Missy" derisively. After living with me for seven years post diagnosis, they say, "Saint Missy" affectionately, but what does that mean about me?

Truthfully, someone who has bipolar disorder is living with a disease that is a bit like playing a game of Russian Roulette. Which side of the bipolar bed am I going to wake-up on today?

And, since it's like that for the person with illness, it's like that for everyone in the house.

Mom has learned how to de-escalate like a champ. Given my younger, much more volatile sister's behavior, (as mad as I have been at her, I've defended her that her disease has control of her brain, therefore, it's not her full self that you're getting) Mom has learned that, if you yell back, you will only escalate the situation.

Dad, on the other hand, is handicapped by his own ADHD and, if he perceives that you're "using him," and "not showing gratitude," he can be pretty vicious. Whereas, he'll simply walk away from Sara because he, like Mom, fear her to some degree. He can be downright cruel to me and expect me, even though Sara and I share disease, to handle things as if I don't have it.

That being said, I wouldn't trade my Mom and Dad for anyone else's parents. They help keep me fed, clothed, and they made sure I was able to attend AOF in 2019. Several times, they stepped up where *Letters to Daniel* is concerned. They got a hotel for a few nights so that I could use their house as a location. I don't pay rent. Usually, I give them the EBT card to help with groceries. They let me hoard it over four months' time so that I can feed my cast and crew.

I don't know how many parents would do all that, but I'm sure they are many like that out there. I try to keep in mind that they take me more seriously now. They understand me, they support me, and they love me. They buy my medications for me so that I can focus on propelling my career forward.

So, when I get mad at them for their inability to read me, I try to remind myself that they're doing their best, and that they do a lot for me. Really, they love our whole family. For example, Sara's vehicle died. They let her use the Versa, (which supposedly was supposed to be mine) she was in a wreck (not her fault), totaled the Versa. They gave her the new Honda to drive. She dented the car with the seatbelt, and the censor was left on, causing the power to drain from the battery. They got it fixed, and she's still using the Honda. And they will buy her a car, eventually, from Isaiah (my nephew).

I'm not trying to trash my sister, she's just really hard on cars, like I'm hard on computers, and shoes.

And thanks to Mom and Dad, while she needs the help, Sara will always have a car. And because of them, while I need it, I will have a place to live, and will be able to pursue my art.

GAYLE SUBLETT: MY FAVORITE EPISCOPALIAN PRIEST

Gayle isn't with us anymore. She contracted tuberculosis as a child and had RA (rheumatoid arthritis) as an adult. She was taking medication for the RA, however, she worked herself like there was no tomorrow. As a priest, she was one of the few whom I felt reflected true service to God, and was what her congregation was about. She's humble. She did not seek to lead a megachurch flock, instead choosing to tend a considerably small flock in Messiah Trinity. Unfortunately, she contracted pneumonia and, very quickly, her already compromised lungs gave out.

The world lost a brilliant light.

I feel that I have to dedicate a chapter to her because, when I returned home from Texas, she was the one who helped me plug into a therapist, and a psychiatrist. In truth, I owe a good part of my recovery to her.

As I staggered and stumbled through treatment for those eighteen months, I wasn't charged a dime, and that was because Gayle got me the hook-up.

As Missy and I started penning scripts again, we needed a place for auditions. Gayle readily offered up Messiah Trinity's reception hall. Gayle was a lot like my memaw, in that she was trying to save my soul.

Although she was just as implacable, she was less judgmental. It was just constant, gentle persistence in inviting me to Sunday service. In her own unobtrusive way, her servant's heart was reaching out to mine.

Little did I know that I would follow a servant's path. Only, I had no desire to serve any organized religion. My flock would be the millions suffering from bipolar disorder and a myriad of other mental illnesses.

I didn't know that while she was, alive, though, that she worked tirelessly to serve her congregation. Even though our congregation was small, its needs were many. And anyone looking to make a full-time salary working as a priest there was really in the wrong place.

There were a few pretenders to the throne. Gayle was a rarity, a female priest. She was an angel among men. As I said, she was always there for you if you needed someone. Did you need a bill paid? She would discuss it with the board, and it would be done. Even if some of the board members were a little tight-fisted at the time, she was always on the side of those in need.

She did not turn away immigrants. If anything, she gathered them up closer to her heart because they needed a champion.

While sharing an apartment with Missy, we found ourselves in the untenable place between starting a new job and paychecks coming in. Gayle spoke to the board. When the board was unmoved, my cousin, Corey, said, "I have $100 in my pocket, if someone will match." That did the trick. The board relented and my rent for that month was paid.

My Aunt Debbie, Aunt Jan, and Uncle Frank always struggle. They are on the razor's edge of having a home and being homeless. The board has voted to assist Debbie and Frank on several occasions.

Gayle was always the driving force behind the generosity of such already good people. When she passed, it was sudden, and it was a shock to us all. None of us really comprehended how sick she really was that winter.

The turnout for her memorial service was a huge testament to how many lives she touched. Much like Missy's Dad, she was well-liked, beloved, and loved. When she died, it left a leadership vacuum at Messiah Trinity.

We bounced from interim priest to interim priest. We didn't have a flashy building ala "Six Flags over Jesus." We didn't have ATMs in our lobby to encourage large tithing. We don't judge the poor. We don't shun people who different from us, we welcome all types.

We're not interested who's going to burn hell; we want to see who we can help the most. That part of Gayle's legacy lives on. And, when I started my long climb out of the bipolar disorder hole, they were there, and they understood why medication was key. They met me with compassion, and not laying the "you can pray it away," or "maybe it's God's will that you have this." (I've been told both, and I just wanted to smack the shit out the people who said it.)

My church doesn't lay on that God wouldn't give you more than you can handle crap on me. God gave me a brain and told me that there are psychiatrists, and therapists, out there. They can give you medicine, and tools, to battle this disease.

In fact, when I needed money for my film and AOF, the donations poured in and added up to over $500. For my church, that is a lot of money. I'm going to have a special screening for them come October. Have everyone cook a pot of chili and make it a potluck.

They invested in me. That is Gayle's legacy in action. Without them neither the film, nor trip, would have happened.

The priest there now, Suzannah, brings her black lab, Sophie, to church every Sunday, or every church event during the week. The dog is my favorite part of when I attend Sunday service. Animals make great service pets and/or emotional support animals.

Messiah Trinity is really two congregations that come together as one so that neither church had to close its doors. One was Lutheran, the other was Episcopal. Together, they are small, but their love and support has been massive.

Gayle was always persuading me to come to church. While I consider Messiah Trinity my church, I should probably give a caveat. I am not a regular Sunday church goer. My sleep cycle is such I am up until late. I drink caffeine late. I pound out the words. You know caffeine turns the slow brain into the one that forms all the words.

Gayle's legacy has made a lasting impact on me.

When I created the blog *Letters to Daniel*, it was just to be an open letter to my favorite actor. But, as I wrote that first letter, I realized that I was trying to cram my life story in the length of one letter. And, second, it dawned on me I was creating a platform that was unique to me. I decided that there was no better person to tell my life story to than *Daniel Craig*, himself. He doesn't know me. Last time I checked, he wasn't even aware that I exist, so I felt free to bare my soul and not worry about having an audience that judged me.

What I couldn't have anticipated was the overwhelming response I received regarding my blog. And as I visited it and wrote regularly, I could feel myself growing stronger, steadier, and more stable. Did I have my detractors? Yes. But I found that, when you begin to rise, people will not only be drawn to your truth, they will come at you to try and tear you down.

My strongest desire is to tour with my movie, (*Letters*) and my books (*Something to Believe In, This One, The Guardian*, and *The Healing Hands Trilogy*) and speak at colleges, universities and, eventually, to medical conventions, and NAMI's national conference. I want to be an advocate because, by sharing my story, I have kept myself honest. Since 2011, I have made great strides, and suffered terrible setbacks, only to rise from the ashes again.

Am I a superwoman who has conquered mental illness? Far from it. I've learned what my limitations are and have learned to ride the wave of symptoms that can, and still do, plague me. I'm just much better at recognizing what the triggers are and how to avoid them.

If I can share the truth of my pain, and my daily recovery process with someone newly diagnosed, it gives them hope. Then, I've done my job. Or, if someone sees their story in mine, and it helps them finally admit they need help, then that makes me feel like I'm doing what I was gifted to do.

Advocacy work, whether it's through my art, or simply sharing my story with people, it is very satisfying. I feel Gayle would have approved.

Considering she worked at Caritas (aka Our Lady of Peace) and connected me with my first mental health professionals in Kentucky, I think that she would be proud. Because when it comes to my mental health, I think, and I believe, that it holds true for my career, too, my guiding light of advocacy in the beginning of my recovery journey was an actor, Maurice Benard. The interesting thing is we're doing a lot of the same things now. He has *State of Mind*. I have *Recovery Unplugged* and *Amy Unplugged*. I've written (if you count this book) three memoirs. He has penned a memoir, and I'm touring to back them. He's touring to promote his.

Albeit, he has a larger platform than I do because his face graces everyone's television on a daily basis; we both have a passion for advocacy work and the arts. And I was hoping this December that I could travel to see him and explain how his willingness to share his story led me to get treatment and how my life has turned around in a major way.

I want to tell him how when I was at my sickest I watched him accept his award and say, "If you have manic depression, and I can do it, then so can you." I want to tell him that I took his message to heart and, now, I want to help others like me. And, even though I don't have mainstream success, I have acquired a following, and I keep grinding like I do in the hope that, one day, I can save lives and create art.

I want to tell him that I've written thirty-one books, and had twenty-seven of them had been published since 2011. I want to tell him I've created twenty-three film projects. I've co-written thirty-three scripts, and that Missy and I have won one hundred and six awards across our body of work since 2014.

And it all starts with wanting to write a script so that we could work together. That led to me questioning my highs and lows, and my hellish mixed episodes. As much as Daniel Craig's work kept me toiling away and sticking with treatment, Maurice was the direct reason I walked into the Center for Health Care Services in San Antonio, Texas and asked to be evaluated for depression, and manic depression. This was before they changed the lingo to bipolar disorder because it is, supposedly, less stigmatizing. It's not. People still have a preconceived notion of what someone with bipolar disorder is like.

What I loved Gayle for, and greatly admire Maurice for, is

their capacity to serve without expectation of getting anything back. But, from what I have learned, when I give, I also receive. I give support and love. Then, I receive support and love. I can no longer tell Gayle how thankful that I am for her, I can only hope that, one day, I will get the chance to tell Maurice.

IN THE HOME STRETCH: 30 DAYS
AND COUNTING

Sometimes, the hardest part is waiting for a finished product. Clint was amazing on the edit. Efficient, fast, and experienced. I loved have my picture ready so quickly. Cleaning up the sound, adding beautiful music that will only elevate the film that everyone has labored so hard and so lovingly on.

I want to take a moment and thank everyone who had a hand in making *Letters to Daniel* a possibility.

And there are many of you. The people behind *Letters to Daniel*, of course, are too many to count. From the successful GoFundMe, and From the Heart Productions campaigns, there were the many generous donations.

I would be remiss if I didn't mention my hard-working, extended cast, some of which I'll be working with again in the second of 2019. I worked with over thirty actors over the course of six days. They gave me their all, and didn't complain once, at least, not within my earshot.

As I reflect on all the circumstances that led up to us finally actually filming *Letters to Daniel*, I feel compelled to give readers who might be considering a life in the film industry some advice.

One, take a good long look at your motivations for wanting to be a part of Hollywood, because you are, most likely, going to be starting off in BFE local film town. I'm in Kentucky and have been kind of unsuccessfully at drawing local talent to my film. But, by traveling to Ohio, Florida, Nevada, Tennessee, and California, I have been able to connect with world class talent to my project. Not that talent doesn't exist in my hometown, or yours, for that matter, but I had a very big falling out with people who were fixtures on the scene, and it led to the closing of some doors.

That's another thing, the cold hard truth is that Hollywood isn't looking to produce your masterpiece of script. You need to start networking at festivals, and grow your base. I built a platform on bestselling books, award-winning scripts, and award winning-documentaries, music videos, trailers, microfilms, and short films.

I wish I could say this all happened overnight, but the reality is that my publishing career didn't start happening until Missy's dad was deteriorating in the hospital. It was the dawning realization that careers don't just happen. That the real work happens after you write the book, writing the synopsis, or synopses, for different agents and publishers.

That's another thing, in the publishing world, you have options. You face a very different landscape than I did. Amazon has taken to treating its self-published writers like crap, especially since so many feel pressured to play their game.

Amazon, when I was getting started, opened its pocketbooks

in a very big way to independent artists. Are we all flocked to Amazon in droves. Great writers, good writers, bad writers, it was a very crowded playing field. The struggle to stand out from your competition was as real then as it is now.

As a writer, you need an editor, a cover artist, and a formatter. If you network right, then you can get those things for free. As an independent filmmaker, it's harder. Films, even at their cheapest, are expensive to make.

To begin with, you need equipment. Even the most basic of stuff will cost you quite a few dollars. Then, there's the software; you can save money there by getting subscriptions. Ten or twenty dollars a month can add up but, screenwriting, much like novel writing, is a long game.

The overnight successes are few and far between. I am forty-four years old. In publishing, there have been ninety-eight-year-olds who had published for the first time. While film is a young male person's game, if you're a woman, and you want it badly enough, then you can have it, and you can have it as long as you keep your eyes on your own lane. This is important as you're reaching to pull yourself up with one hand, be sure that the other is extended back down to help those coming up behind you.

During my twenties, I had no one in a position of experience willing to help me and Missy. When I got sick, it was as if I had the black plague. People believe that bipolar disorder is contagious, and that is simply load of crap. However, it's the most natural repellent you could ever ask for.

While people are talking more openly about depression and bipolar disorder now, there is still a strong stigma attached to it. And Hollywood is like any other industry when it comes to addressing these ills.

Especially passionate people in positions of power get films about mental illness made. *Shine* is a good example, starring Geoffrey Rush. Or *A Beautiful Mind*, starring Russell Crowe quite possibly Ron Howard's modern day classic. Some say that *Rain Man* is a good example, but I disagree, as that movie isn't about Dustin Hoffman's character, but Tom Cruise's.

Film analysis aside, people are going to want to put you in a box and label you. As for me, it was first, the marketer, locally. Slowly, it has become mental health advocate. I don't ever know if they'll see me as talented artist, but that's something I obsess about less and less these days.

If you want to be a writer/director in Hollywood, then you will have to hone your craft, as well as network. You will have to go where the connections are. And, quite probably, you will either have to produce/direct your passion project, or you will have to connect with someone who is as just as excited to produce your script as you are.

Another thing you will find is, that if you network right, you can get people, who want to sign on to your vision. If your script is great, and you believe in your vision, and you build a brand around that vision, then things will start to happen for you.

I had several paternalistic men talk down to me and tell me, "As long as you insist on directing your script, it will never get made." A well-known producer/director in the faith-based industry said it to me rather dismissively, and a director was an absolute dick about.

I met with several so-called producers who just wanted to be paid while you do all the work. As I soldiered on, it came down to this: *How badly did I want it?*

Did I want it badly enough to go all in? To, somehow, get enough seed money to get it off the ground and be willing to sacrifice everything? Sleep, sanity, money? To, somehow, take all my talents and bring them to bear on my dream of a film? Did I have it in me to pull off the hardest thing that I had ever done?

Well, you know the answer to that by now. The movie will screen privately at my parents' church as a thank you. And test screen at Imaginarium.

Letters to Daniel was born as a blog six years ago, a script in 2015. Some films take much longer to see come to fruition, some shorter. It's just an example of independent filmmaking being a long game.

I published first in 2011. Eight years ago. I'd learned a lot about writing, and editing, that I was able to apply to my screenplays.

When you're an artist, you're always learning, and I learned a lot from Mark and Clint. They're wonderful collaborators, as well as great mentors. Their willingness to show me the ropes, give sage advice, and still allow me to create my film as I saw fit, served to boost my confidence in a big way.

Still the movie would had never been made had the actors and crew not agreed to work for little more the gas, food, in some cases shelter, and an IMDb credit.

I want to say I am proud of how the film has turned out so far. All that is left is for Valyo to work on the sound edit and what I am sure is going to be a beautiful score. He has been influenced heavily by Alan Silvestri (he composed the score for *Forrest Gump*), and he has already composed the intro to the film.

To say I was on pins and needles was an understatement. It was a bit like waiting to unwrap my presents at Christmas. The anticipation was as great as a child that you hoped that the actuality of the present didn't disappointment you. But, unlike presents, Valyo's gift as a musician is amazing.

I believe that the angels above sing when his music is played.

The one thing I wanted the first composer I worked with to know is that I made a choice based on the music in Valyo's music library that I had the privilege of hearing. It's not that my first composer wasn't talented, it was that Valyo, at least at that point, could elevate the value of my films.

The two of us have similar goals. His end game is to land in Hollywood as an in demand composer. His music matches the emotional tone of my films. As long as I can use him I will.

However, for my next project, the suspense-thriller, I decided that I'm going with Ricardo Raymundo, mostly because Valyo doesn't compose for horror. Not anymore. So, for this film, it's Ricardo.

As I wait I try to fill my time with other projects. Such as editing the trailer. I'm going to work on it some more tomorrow. I'm working on the shot list for HOME. To be filmed in November.

I'd like to thank Mysti Parker, and family, once more, for hosting my cast and crew. It's not easy to give up your home, even if you are being compensated.

I'd also like to thank the businesses that hosted *Letters to Daniel*: OG Auto, Christy Cox, MD and Associates, the Ramada Plaza and Conference Center, Village 8 Movie Theaters, Messiah Trinity Church, my Mom and Dad, Air BnB host and hostess in Germantown, and my Aunt Debbie and Aunt Jan and Uncle Frank, you are all beautiful people and businesses and without you my dream wouldn't have come true.

I wish to address the volatile nature of mine and my sister, Sara's, relationship. I may bitch about her, wish like hell that she did things differently, but she's sick, not evil. When I'm mad, I tend to forget that. Bipolar disorder does ugly things to people.

Sara, at her best, is a big-hearted, loving, sensitive, generous, mother, and sister. She feels things deeply, as I do. Only, she's not getting proper treatment, but that does not make her any less deserving of love and compassion. Sometimes, I just have to keep my distance so that I don't get triggered. But, Sara, if you're reading this, I do love you.

STARVING IN TEXAS

*T*wenty years ago, had you told me that I would be making a film about Missy's and my struggles with my mental illness, I would have said, "You're crazy." But, now, my work is littered with my thoughts on mental illness and how society, at large, responds to it. Twenty years ago, Missy and I were about to head out for Texas and, had I known then what I know now about bipolar disorder, perhaps that adventure would have never happened.

One night, we were sitting on my parents' couch, and Missy said, "What are you feeling, just write it down."

I took the legal pad and proceeded to write, *"die, die, die, die."*

Missy did, and still does, take this as a deliberate attempt on my part to hurt her. Nothing could be further from the truth.

We kept insane hours during the summer of 1999 before we left for San Antonio. She worked part-time at UPS, full-time at B. Dalton's. Then, there were the all-nighters with me penning screenplays. In 1999, we went from reading and editing each other's work to writing together.

One night, as she crashed and burned, I felt so abandoned, and so alone, that I started to cry, hard, as if I was the last person on earth. I felt as alone as ever.

In retrospect, that should have been a huge, waving red flag indicating that I needed to get some help.

Another thing that should have tipped me off was that I was getting less and less sleep. I would lie down at 6:00 a.m., jacked up on RC and Cherry Pull n' Peels, and mind would race. I couldn't slow down, or relax.

Hindsight being what it is, I might have been better served staying put in Kentucky but, then, I wouldn't have been gifted with the *Letters to Daniel* project. And with it all kinds of personal growth. And sort of franchise that has seen me through incredible opportunities and setbacks only to be gifted with opportunities again.

In the beginning our time in Texas was a trial by fire. We had very little money. Our grocery list consisted of things like spaghetti, peanut butter, and hot dogs, three things I have a hard time stomaching these days. It may not have been ideal, but living on ramen was better than starving to death. The ironic thing was, even though we were hardly eating, we were packing on the pounds. It was in part because of the medication I was taking and in part because we were eating processed foods.

Breakfast consisted of, one egg, one slice of bacon, and a piece of toast. Lunch, a peanut butter, or bologna, sandwich, pretzels, and soft drinks, or water. And supper was either spaghetti, or hot dogs.

That was the menu, all day, every day.

Snacks including popcorn, and generic Kool-Aid. I can't eat popcorn now because of diverticulitis, but Kool-Aid is something I cannot abide by. Capri-Suns yes. Cola, Oh, yes! But Kool-Aid, no.

Twenty dollars was usually our limit yet, sometimes, we wanted an entertainment magazine, and that made for an even tighter budget, which meant more processed food instead of healthy choices.

And, even though we were walking everywhere, we were gaining weight, especially me.

That hardly seemed fair. But that was the reality of taking powerful meds and eating poorly.

My Aunt Rosie was down there for a few months. She took us out to KFC, Mi Tierra's, and the local cultural custom of Las Posadas. In the film, Ginny mispronounces the custom. What it consists of is the community (of Catholics) gathering together at the MACC (Mexican-American Cultural Center). Everyone is given candles, they were supposed to be lit, but the wind was blowing so hard that we just carried the candles.

Everyone walked throughout the neighborhood with a man and a woman going from do to door, the man playing guitar, and the two of them singing as Mary and Joseph, asking for a place to stay. Every participating home owner responding that it didn't matter what their name was and would proceed to turn them away, until the last house where they would be welcomed inside.

At the end, we went back to the MACC and had Mexican cocoa, which is gelatinous, and bitter, compared to hot chocolate in the United States. There were also tasty light, pastries. All in all, it was a delightful time. Being exposed to a culture different from my own proved to be one of the most rewarding things I'd experienced in San Antonio.

It was fun to walk with the community and not feel so isolated, for once. The bipolar disorder had definitely left me feeling like the odd man out, like I was wearing the scarlet letters *MD*, for manic depression so that the world could judge me.

Having Aunt Rosie there was something of a Godsend. She helped us survive those first few brutal months. She introduced us to the story of Our Lady of Guadalupe, and we watched the telenovela that she had been instructed to watch while she was at the MACC. She was perfecting her conversational Spanish so that she could better serve the Centro Latino community when she returned to Kentucky.

Before she left for Kentucky, she took us to Mi Tierra's one last time. In the film, it is a coffeehouse because we could not get a Mexican restaurant to cooperate with us. It ended up being a very nice location that we were able to use for two scenes.

The owner of the location turned the music down for us so that we didn't run into right issues with the film, which was very kind of them. Had they been busy, we would have represented a massive disruption to business for them. As it was, most of their customers opted for the drive-thru.

When Missy and I were in Texas we had to get creative with our audition spaces. The first time, we used an office space in the front of the apartment complex we had been living at the time. The second round of auditions were held in the meeting room of the local library.

During the callbacks, one actor we had pegged for the role of J said of another character, "Some of the things she says kind of hurt my feelings," to which everyone laughed. The role of Gemini in *You're the Reason* is funny but, in lesser actor's hands, she could be reduced to a one-dimensional bitch.

The ironic thing is that nearly every actress we came across said, "I am Gemini!" Even my cousin, Crystal, said it before she read for her. Alas, the film is not meant to be. I hate that Missy turned J into the bad guy at the expense of the integrity of the character of Gemini. She didn't intend to, but I refuse to shop it, or film it.

Is that a bitchy thing to do? Probably. It was supposed to be our first feature. That was back in 1999. The rewrite in 2013 was a solid script, but we've become better writers since then. And my feelings on the matter remain unmoved. I'm mad at how it turned out, so I have no desire to waste my time and film it.

On the upside is that we have continued to create more viable, and better-scripted, material. But, while we were in Texas, it was basically our calling card script. And, even in its original form, it needed work. The 2013 version would eventually bring us an award at the International Indie Gathering.

When I view my work too harshly, it serves me well to remember that TIG draws world class talent to their screenwriting competition. The likes of Jason Tostevin, JoAnn Hess, and Bob Messinger are Indie Hall of Famers.

I do my best to learn what I can from each of those people. God knows that there is a lot of knowledge in that Holy Trinity of writers. It's very nice that I've had the privilege of becoming friends with two of them. I'm not as close to JoAnn, but Bob has become someone whom I talk to every day, and it helps to ally my anxiety.

Every day, I wake up, and the battle to push passed to the anxiety of the blank page is very real. To go from script to screen requires a bit of magic, and writing is the most powerful magic of all. Because, without the ability to write, there is no eventual cinema, none worth watching, in my opinion.

I mean, talk shows and reality television have their place; one of my projects is in development is actually a talk show. But fiction provides an escape, a chance to heal and dream of possible new adventures for yourself.

The magic of the movies, at least in creating them, is that you are provided with an opportunity to collaborate and grow as an artist in a way you can't when working solo.

When working on *Letters to Daniel*, every last crew member taught me some valuable lessons about what and what not to do. The actors showed me what being vulnerable in front of the camera is all about.

Shooting *Letters to Daniel*, I was worlds away from Texas in many ways. I was not forced to live in the world of the starving artist, though, in a way, we are all starving artists in the independent world. I'm not worried about where my next meal is coming from. I'm not worried about going naked. And, for the foreseeable future, I know that I will have the support of my family, to be able to pursue my passions as I see fit.

For now, I am left to create in my own sandbox, without the intrusion of haters and those few who resent me for being me. (They are out there.) And wait for the finished file from Valyo.

I have heard some samples of Valyo's work and I can't wait to hear the rest of what he has to offer. The submissions process will begin in earnest next month. To both big and small festivals to give it a chance at wide distribution.

Upliftv, (cable) Parables, (Roku) and their parent company, Olympusat, wants *Letters to Daniel*. So does NAMI (National Alliance for the Mentally Ill). And there are some other avenues, like possibly being on airliners, and a former major movie studio executive wants to review it.

I am blessed to be what feels like on a seismic shift in mine and Missy's career. I feel like I have taken a step forward, and Missy and I have hit the anvil repeatedly over these past eight years and with some luck, the final cut of *Letters to Daniel* will open some long closed doors.

I can't wait for *Letters to Daniel* to screen for its first audience and officially be out to the world. It will have made starving in Texas worth it.

WHY MISSY AND MY CAT WILL
ALWAYS BE #1

My sister, Sara, and I had a discussion once that upset her mightily. (We tend to do that a lot to each other.) She contends that I always put my friends above her, and the rest of the family. That's a gross generalization. I'm good to my friends. I'm open about who I am with them, and they respect me for being a hardworking, creative person trying to burst through to the mainstream. And the feeling is mutual.

She says that my friendships are more important to me than, say, she is. Or, Brandy. Or Mom and Dad. I wouldn't say that; people whom I call my friends are few and far between. As rule, I have a better caliber of friend than Sara does. This is not a reflection of Sara's character, she's always been a better friend to her friends than they have been to her. That being said, there were exceptions.

But I have friends who, in the end, are more like family, and I'm sure that I have some industry friends, should I suddenly stop creating, who would disappear, that if I could no longer help them would have nothing to do with me. However, I have my support network, Missy, Mom, and Dad. Luke (my cat). I also have my creative life.

My creative life is teeming with the kind of support that I could only dream about during my early twenties. Writing is my meditation, and my escape. Directing and producing are harder, so people who help me in that end are going to get some love, too.

Now, that doesn't mean I love my family any less; I take exception to that. Would I say that there's a strain to mine, and my blood sisters', relationships, the honest answer is, "Yes." I could have been accused of not reaching out to bridge that gap when, on countless occasions, I have. I'd just gotten tired of reaching to get no response.

What it boils down to is that I live a life and have a lifestyle that neither Sara, nor Brandy, understand. I get heavy resentment from Sara, I guess, because life for her is always stressful, volatile, and a financial scramble.

Life is basically stress, and my stress is not her stress. She's raising two boys without their father. My mother and father are saints. She leans heavily on them but, then, they let a lot of people lean heavily on them.

As for my cat, Luke is the fourth cat I've considered mine. Chyna was with me for nearly fourteen years, and she was an orange tabby. Runt of the litter, so wild that she bordered on feral. But, every winter, she would snuggle under the blankets and keep me warm. She passed away just as me and Missy were starting to make a name for ourselves on the festival circuit.

Luke is also an orange tabby but, obviously, a he. He is not the runt. He is a big fat tomcat who likes to sleep on my computer which sits on my desk next to my head at night. Sometimes, he sits on my feet when I'm writing in the recliner, or curled up on my bed next to me when I write at my desk.

Sara accuses me of loving my friends more than her. No, I love my cat more than anyone. He knows when I am sad or "out of sorts." He knows when I need him and, if I'm crying, he comes running up to me and gives me whisker kisses.

Luke doesn't judge me, have any expectations of me, or demands anything me. He only wants to be fed and have his litter box cleaned. Humans are much more complicated, and messy. Animals have emotions, too, but I feel that humans expect a thriving friendship, and a close relationship, when they've done little to nothing to earn it.

Sara wants me to treat her the way I treat Missy. I have to laugh because I don't think she fully comprehends what that means.

I love Missy. She's the sister that I always wanted, and we came to be in one another's lives by chance. She was working at a bookstore, and I was the last hire-in for Christmas help. The odds were not good that I would be kept on, let alone that Missy and I would form a lifelong friendship, and creative partnership, from our time together there.

For a year, we were simply friends at work. I wouldn't really say friends, because I didn't really call her outside of work, go to dinner with her, or see movies with her. We weren't even writing together during that first year. We each worked on our individual projects and brought them to work so the others could critique them. So, before we were anything else, we were each other's beta readers. Or, in Missy's case, she told her stories orally because she was afraid to hand her actual work over to me.

Even so, Missy's initial impression of me was that I was a bit crazy, and that I was crazy because I talked about my life (being sexually abused) in such a bold, and open, manner. Granted, neither one of us knew that I had bipolar disorder at the time but, in retrospect, it was obvious to anyone who knew me that I swung high and low, without the volatile nature that often comes with bipolar disorder. That wouldn't show itself until further down the road, when Missy and I landed in Texas, and the pressures became too much to bear.

We worked together a year before the idea of writing together ever was brought up. What started out as a couple of days a week writing quickly snowballed into nightly phone calls and, pretty soon, nightly write-ins on a dreadful novel which we birthed. What we salvaged from it were the twin girl characters, Ariel and Adriana Stuart, heirs to a criminal empire. Fueled by Big Red, RC, Twizzlers and, on one dicey occasion Vivarin, we created the sprawling novel, for which when we ran out of plot, we just added a character. When we killed our first character off, we cried. When we killed our second character off, we couldn't stop laughing, which either says something about us and how weird we really are, or something about the writing.

Missy fatefully proposed that move to San Antonio in the summer of 1999 when we were both having difficulties at home. I chalk it up to growing pains and mental illness and the very real need to separate from our parents.

That, in and of itself, is very stressful. At that time, she was the only person whom I trusted completely. To be absolutely honest, she still is. I have that haunting fear that, given the chance, my well-intentioned mom would lock me away should the waters get rough.

I have people whom I confide in other than Missy. They are few and far between, but they are there. But the fact remains that, when Missy and I were alone and isolated in San Antonio facing down poverty and hunger and stigma, she remained with me, and never left my side. Given how bumpy the ride was, she would have been completely justified in bailing. But whatever her reasons were for sticking around, (she says it was because I was getting help and was trying to get better) the fact is that she did remain.

When we moved back to Kentucky on the eve of the 2000 election, it felt like defeat. Dealing with me in that particular head space was no treat. The reality was that I was spiraling down, and rapid cycling, while we searched for the right drug cocktail. With psychiatry, and the treatment of bipolar disorder, it really is part art, and part science.

I would rage out of control. Missy was on the front line, very much alone in her fight to help keep me from going off the rails. Dealing with me borderline unhinged is no treat. But, indeed, it was a testament to what we were both going through.

Inside my head was chaotic mess and, somehow, Missy found a way to weather the bipolar storm and help us become stronger for it.

Initially, my return brought with it humble pie, defeat, and the inability to trust my family. They couldn't understand why I didn't, and I wasn't able to full articulate why. It boiled down to me being angry at being forced to move back to the Kentucky. No movie. No contacts. No success. What had I gotten while down there? A proper diagnosis and partial treatment.

I knew the return to home base was necessary but I was, and can be, an all or nothing girl. I used to set myself up for failure this way all the time, but adjusting to life back in Kentucky was hard.

I had to admit the life I had imagined for myself was not going to come to pass. I needed to circle the wagons, lean on my support network, take my meds, and get into therapy. But, even in the thick of giving up at the bottom, I found that I still could dream. And those dreams I was dreaming could still come true, but I had to get well; I had to get stable for any of it to happen, and I had to readjust to what success really meant in my life.

So, when I say that I put Luke as my number one that doesn't mean other people do not have a place in my heart, and my life. It just means that Luke makes no demands on me. He loves me unconditionally. Humans love conditionally. At least, it has been my experience that they do.

My mom says that she loves unconditionally, but she expects a certain amount of love in return. And that's fair; she's my mom, and I love her. But I expect her, (sometimes to my disappointment), to respect me like she respects my sister, Brandy.

I think the only caveat to this for the human race is that they have the capacity to love grandchildren and fur-babies unconditionally. But, even then, not everybody has that capacity. Because people are only human, and humans are flawed and are prone to acts of selfishness. Only God can truly love unconditionally.

Missy is the one person whom I feel like I come closest to loving unconditionally. That's why Missy and Luke will always be my number ones, next to God.

33

BRUSHES WITH GREATNESS:
CINDY BOND

*I*n 2018, I went to see the film *I Can Only Imagine*, a Mission Studios International production starring Dennis Quaid. In May 2018, I also attended ICFF.

I maneuvered it alone; it was overwhelming. Not because it was the biggest festival I'd been to, but because people aren't naturally inclined to work with one another. Sure, there is a pecking order there, and they do things like a dinner, and what not. But, even if you get into the film festival, you have to pay for a film pass to get you into the screenings and the seminars even after your project gets selected for screening.

The unintentional stigmatization there was massive. I encountered it everywhere I turned, especially from well-meaning filmmakers and producers. People said such damaging things as God wanted you to go through this so you could help other people like you. Then, why do all the other people have to suffer? It's awfully arrogant to believe God would single me out to lead the masses.

I believe that God gave us the intelligence to use psychiatrists, and therapists, in our quest to get better, and to stabilize. He provides us with people in our lives to help support us in our day to day struggle. Bipolar disorder is an illness, not a death sentence, and not a curse from the Devil proving you're too flawed for God's love.

At another festival, a festival I love, (not AOF), a gentleman informed me that, maybe, God doesn't mean for you to be healed from bipolar disorder. I wanted to punch him dead in his mouth.

If he was the one with the disease, then he would realize what a cruel and narrow-minded assessment that is, as it is he wanted to talk scripture. When he threw the Old Testament in my face, I threw the New Testament in his. The conversation ended with that.

IF people truly followed the word of God, then they would be a kind, loving, and inclusive faith. What you have is all these factions who believe they are the definitive answer when it comes to what God wants for this world?

While I was at this festival, I met some nice people who, if I look at their Facebook pages, I would lose my lunch at what they believe politically. But, at a film festival, I believe that the art is what should be talked about.

The problem I have with faith-based films is there is little concern about the art. They are so, excuse the expression, hell bent on getting their message across they don't concern themselves with production value. The message is usually crammed down your throat in a forced conversion experience.

I mean, the movies look nice, sound nice, but the acting, and writing, p-u.

I mentioned that I went to see *I Can Only Imagine* before I attended the festival. It is about the lead singer of Mercy Me's inspiration behind the song behind the hit single.

It's a beautiful song. And, when I went to see the movie with Missy, I related to the lead singer's character. His father was a cold, unfeeling, bastard who abused him, and when he's dying they mend fences. When he passes on, the song is born.

I cried hard during this film. I don't foresee me and my biological father ever mending fences, not for lack of effort on my part. He's forever spitting on my dreams, and the way I go about achieving them. Needless to say, *I Can Only Imagine* touched a nerve, and it was a cathartic experience.

Did it magically fix things with my biological father? Not even close. But it was one of the better faith based-films that I'd ever seen.

At ICFF, Cindy Bond was a special guest. She was forever moving from one place to another. But, as I was leaving the restaurant, I ran smack into her and asked if could have a few minutes of her time.

I told her about *Letters to Daniel*'s pedigree. She got on Amazon, and ordered the print book; we discussed it over lunch. She was warm, friendly, and attentive. I felt as if she were really listening to me and taking me seriously.

She told me to send her the script, and that she would take it under advisement. Mission Pictures International has a partnership with theaters in the United States, and does global distribution.

Cindy was also the main producer on *I Can Only Imagine*, which broke all kinds of box office records. As much as I liked the film, it wasn't nearly as gritty, as I'd hoped it would be. In truth, faith-based movies are rarely raw, gritty, and real. They tend not to soft pedal and sugarcoat.

As I talked to Cindy, I realized that *Letters to Daniel* might not be an exact fit, but I plowed ahead, anyway, with my pitch and, by the end of it, I had her email contact information.

211

Well, upon arrival back home, I emailed everything that she had requested of me. Then, I proceeded to wait for a month and a half. The waiting was like being water boarded, and slowly waiting for the best of everything, or the worst of everything.

In June, I got the worst of everything. It read, *"While your story is inspiring it's not quite the right fit. We researched our international markets and it shows they want romantic dramas..."* Blah blah blah. *"Feel free to retry when the film is finished."* Blah blah blah.

It seems to be our one outside shot at theatrical distribution. Our film is one hour, one minute, and thirty-three seconds long. Usually, they want seventy minutes, or longer. Like I said, it's an outside shot, but we're going to go for it.

I wasn't shocked at the rejection, and I wasn't really mad about it. We live and work in a risk adverse industry. There aren't a lot of spec scripts by newly minted screenwriters being produced in Hollywood these days, though a really great script can get you everything from a paid gig, to representation. But, rarely, are those scripts made by big studios.

The industry waits for the indie to take all the risk, and the hope is that everyone will reap the big rewards of profit. For our $6,000.00 film to look and sound as good as it does is a miracle. I had amazing people on my film.

I hope Mission Pictures International will consider a sixty-one minute film. It would probably be wise to get in touch with Cindy to see if she remembers me. They said, "No" to making it, but it is my hope that we can break through to the mainstream.

Cindy was super nice. And, now that we've proven ourselves, I hope that doors are going to open for us. It would be nice if one of those doors was Mission Pictures International.

I recently received the sound edited sound file for *Letters to Daniel*. Valyo is a fucking genius. What he did was amazing. He balanced the onset audio with the voice over so now there isn't such a disparity between the two.

The dialogue was clear as a bell, and the ambient sound is much less intrusive. I knew that he could do it. But, when Mark and Clint panicked, it gave me pause. Mark listened to part of it and was bowled over. We have been blessed throughout this journey. Valyo is humble, too. He said, "I didn't do anything, it was all in the software." But I explained to him that you have to have the knowledge to apply those filters in the correct way.

To put things into perspective, a lot of people make their husband, or wife, their number one. Some choose to make their children their number one. Others still, they choose their brother or sister.

I have three younger sisters, and one older brother. Each of them have faced their own challenges, have at least been in a serious long-term relationship, if not married, and all have at least one child.

Now, I've had two long term romantic relationships. They happened during my early twenties. They had their good points and, for a time, I maintained friendships with both of them. But, soon, their negative attributes took over where our friendships were concerned.

One had a propensity for dating, and marrying, jealous, if not psychotic in some cases, women. Eventually, the things they said that were too much for me to take. Although, I highly suspect that the estranged wife had something to do with it. It really doesn't matter, for my own mental health, I needed to be done with him.

The other one was never much of a "man," more like a "momma's boy" or "man-child" and, during my early twenties, I was not always stable. He was the weaker of the two of us, but what he did for me was make sex okay to enjoy after suffering abuse as a child, and I learned that I didn't need anyone to believe me, or validate me, to make my memories of what happened true. So he was really wonderful for those two things. Eventually, he moved on, and I did, too. I was too volatile, and he was too vanilla.

Now, why on earth would I have made either one of those young men my number one? Your number one, you have to know, or at least trust, to have your back. As much as I wanted those romantic partners to be worthy of being my number one, they weren't.

Brandy and I were often odds growing up. We ran in very different with very different circles; she was a part of the popular crowd.

Sara, as mad and crazy as she makes me, she had it rough as the youngest in our household. She was five years younger than me, and three and half years younger than Brandy. We often left her out of our playtime and would do things just to get her in trouble. Her mental illness manifested itself at a much younger age, so she had a lot to deal with.

The fact remains, as close as I wish my siblings and I were, we aren't as close as my mom wished us to be. I mean, I love them and, if they need me, I'm totally there. But, as for career and what I do with my time, we just don't travel in the same circles.

As for Sabrina and Kevin, while not close, I try to stay in touch. They, and Brandy, are the only good things my father ever did produce, and he isn't responsible for how well they all turned out.

Missy came into my life right before it all went to shit for a while, and she quite literally saved my life in more ways than one. They say you can't choose who you're related, too. When I was in a tailspin, Missy was there for what was the war of attrition for my soul, and she never gave up. Missy fought, tooth and nail, for me to get into treatment. She gave me an ultimatum get help.

I listened to her. Really, at the time, I had no choice. It was either get help, or die. And, if I hadn't listened to Missy, things like the meeting with Cindy Bond, and the opportunities presenting themselves to me, would not be happening.

34

WHY IMAGINARIUM IS SO
IMPORTANT TO KENTUCKY

*W*hen you're struggling to make it in the arts, whether it's as a musician, a writer, or a film-maker, there's something to be said for having a local community to lean on. Locally, there are great indie filmmakers, and writers. But they're broken up into factions, and everybody does not love everybody. I certainly don't. I'm not privy to the local scene. I may not love everybody, but I do support, and cheer on, everyone's creative endeavors. I don't actively hate anyone in the community. Am I wary of some people? Yes. Am I bewildered by some of their actions against me? Yes.

Let me give you an example. In 2016, a cinematographer offered to help me and Missy. But when given the budget, and the time frame, they backed out, citing that they held themselves to a high level of quality. And we felt that we were kidding ourselves of we thought we could. And, for that reason, they had to bow out.

Fast forward three years. We could, we did and, now, we have a kick ass film because of it. Am I mad at these people? Of course not. Their concerns were legitimate. But, during those years between 2016 and 2019, we picked up some powerful allies who were on the same page as Missy and me. We were a little more seasoned, and we had a magnificent cast and crew.

Another example, a local filmmaker, whom we met at Imaginarium, expressed his support of me and Missy and offered us the use of his studio. We would check in with one another from time to time. Then, about a week after me and Missy and our team filmed *Letters to Daniel*, he contacted me and savagely attacked me, saying that I made my movie on charity and government money, and that I owed him a debt of gratitude. Now, he did bupkiss to support *Letters to Daniel*. Last time I checked, disability is funded by what I had paid into it. He implied that I didn't need it. I crowdfunded, but a lot of indie films are financed through crowdfunding. He said that he owned *Letters to Daniel*, that he owned his own shit because it was on his credit card.

It stung and hurt, but I blocked him, to say the least. Am I mad at him? No. It must be miserable to live in a headspace like that all the time. There's really very little joy to be had. What kind of quality do his films have? Well, it's not cool to trash another artist's work. So I won't say anything on this subject.

I wouldn't say that Imaginarium is a filmmaker's mecca. I would say that Imaginarium is a writer's comic con. At least, that's the direction it's been taking. And, this year, it's taken a huge step in that direction. Context used to be the go-to was a writer's comic con. The film festival is quaint. It draws an eclectic mix, usually, mostly horror, sci-fi, and fantasy (dystopian). The occasional mystery, or drama, but mostly aforementioned genres.

There had been a writer's retreat run by the Green River Writers, and they had a lot of respectable agents, and writers, come through there. While Imaginarium hasn't had any big names, agent wise, come through their doors, they have a solid reputation with reputable small presses, and indie writers.

Missy likes to tell me that I'm worthy of being an Imaginator, and my resume only supports that notion. But I doubt that I'll ever be asked to be an Imaginator, until New York and Hollywood one comes calling. They people in charge just don't see me as a drawing card. But this is the first Imaginarium I'll be teaching a workshop at. On thriving creatively while coping with serious mental illness. I'll be launching three books. And *Letters to Daniel* will get a sneak preview there. Plus an after party. I'll probably have to prepare all the food or buy it at least. All my cash is tied up in the filming of HOME, my suspense-thriller.

Imaginarium was the first place to screen the proof of concept version *Letters to Daniel*. And, although I was in a terrible headspace that Sunday evening in September of 2014, I am fully appreciative of the runner-up award I received. The rules state they have the right not to give an award if they don't see fit, and they had a really good line up of judges that year.

So, out of all my Imaginarium awards, that's one of the two that I'm proudest of. The other is for Best Non-Genre Short Film for our micro *Letters to Daniel: Awareness*. Again, that year, they had an awesome line up of judges. Meaning, had I not won anything those two years, then I would have been perfectly happy knowing I had been judged by people who understood my message and felt that my films were award worthy. In other words, people who had business judging such material.

Imaginarium is important to the state of Kentucky because it's the only major writing convention that makes itself accessible to the public. The prices went up this year. I hope it's a gamble that pays off. Still, even with prices raised it's a nice festival but they have priced my parents out of attending. They were going to come see *Letters to Daniel*, but I couldn't sponsor them (Imaginarium). My career is expanding in such a way that I need to invest in my dream. We will support them with a friend of Imaginarium sponsorship, but the days of breaking myself for Imaginarium are probably over.

That doesn't mean that I don't appreciate, or care about, Imaginarium. They were among the earliest supporters of *Letters to Daniel*. Stephen Zimmer loves his festival, and he loves seeing, and greeting, writers from all over.

Kentucky doesn't have much to offer in terms in advancing a writer's career, beyond the independent scene. Imaginarium is a great place to start as a writer. You can get your feet wet, ask questions, an even pitch your manuscript to a small press, or attend panels, or workshops, that tell you the ins and outs of self-publishing. Some of the guests who have attended are USA Today/NYT Bestseller Robyn Peterman Zahn, and JM Madden. Harlequin Romance Queen, Elizabeth Bevarly. Even Horror King, Brian Keene, has been a guest of honor.

Writing wise, it's tough to beat Imaginarium's line-up. But, when it comes to filmmakers, the guest list is a little lacking, and is a bit lopsided when it comes to the types of films that they create. Not that they're not talented, they just stick mostly to sci-fi, horror, or paranormal and ghost stories.

To wit, on the distribution front a team that does the paranormal thing was on a panel with me about distribution. Now, I have never been to the AFM, (the American Film Market) but I do know a thing or two about distribution by having secured deals for four of my films. Was I rich? No, but this guy and his wife were obnoxious. They were very dismissive of me, and I was like, "Okay, I can either fight this, or let him babble on. I chose to fight it.

He's created a whole persona with his films, and documentaries, and he bragged on himself, which was totally unbecoming. He's not a bad person, but he rubbed me the wrong way.

However, one year, I was on a screenwriting panel with a legit star of screenwriting, Jeffrey Reddick, creator of the *Final Destination* franchise. He was story supervisor for a television series based on a Charlaine Harris (*True Blood*) series. Among many other wonderful accolades, he's very forthcoming on tips for the craft of screenwriting, but he's bit more opaque when it comes to showing his hand on how to get hired by a studio, or securing some representation.

Still, he is a genuinely nice guy, and very approachable for fans and fellow screenwriters, at various levels, on the journey. Without Imaginarium, Jeffery Reddick might come to Kentucky via a Comic Con, such as Lexington's Toy Comic Con, but he wouldn't available for a drink at the bar, or dinner, after panels.

He's the guest of honor this year, returning to Imaginarium after a five year absence. Stephen Zimmer has cultivated a valuable friendship and connection with him. Turns out Jeffery is from Berea, Kentucky. Chances are his connection can't help me, but I still want him to attend the screening of my film. If he likes it, maybe he'll get a drink or come to the after party.

And who knows if he likes the film enough he'll ask if he can show to his executive friends or his agent. But those are all very big ifs. As it is, it would be nice just to have him touched or moved by it.

Imaginarium is important in Kentucky. Residents of the state don't have much in the way of access to the next level if they are aspiring writers, not enough so that people will show them the ropes. Even when someone does do it, there is perhaps a feeling of an asshole hiding behind a nice persona. Imaginarium was born when Lee Martindale was breaking bread with Stephen, and she told him that he needed to create a convention for writers.

Stephen took that to heart because a lot of writers were getting the shaft at Fandom Fest, and not all the writers were a good fit at Conglomeration. Not that Stephen didn't appreciate Fandom Fest, but the writers' portion of that Comic Con got zero support from its creators. I don't want to badmouth them; Ken and Myra do a lot with charity work and have a certain amount of support among filmmakers locally.

But, talk to an indie author at Imaginarium, and you'll get a much different response about Stephen, and Imaginarium. Everyone loves Stephen. And, for the most part, I believe that Stephen wants to see writers and filmmakers succeed in Kentucky.

While Imaginarium is a great regional convention, I think that it's still finding its legs. It's yet to fully blossom. But 2019 had marked something of a turning point for them: more sponsors, bigger sponsors, like ISA, and Spalding University.

Imaginarium is important to Kentucky because writers are often the odd man out. In 2019, Stephen had invited voice actors, podcasters, and a former HBO executive who marketed the *L-Word* when it was on television. I might approach her. Letters to Daniel isn't L-Word but it is a story of female friendship, loyalty, and love. I'm glad that there is an Imaginarium because the actors who live close by (Ohio, a handful of KY actors, and Tennessee) can see the film's premiere without having to travel a long distance or spend a lot of money.

Imaginarium is important to me and Missy because the festival director, Stephen Zimmer, was the first person to give us a seat at the professional creative's table. The lessons I learned writing and selling books have me well in my film career as well.

Ultimately, Imaginarium is what you make of it. And, if you want to use to start your writing career, then you're exactly where you need to be.

35

DANIEL CRAIG AND THE STIRRINGS
OF A DREAM

I've often been asked, "How did you conceive of the "Dear Daniel" blog, and the subsequent memoir, documentaries, microfilms, and trailers all leading up to the script and narrative feature film?" I've also been asked, "Did you plan all this?" *Letters to Daniel* all happened because I wanted to thank the inspiration of many of my heroes. I wanted to thank him for indirectly helping me break through in the publishing world. So I did what any fangirl would do, I created blog and set about writing Daniel an open letter of gratitude.

As I did so, I realized that I was trying to cram thirty-seven plus years of life into a finite letter. So, about halfway through I realized that I could relate my memoirs in that fashion and not feel so self-conscious about putting my life and recovery, as it were, on blast.

The first letter was about thanking Daniel Craig. In a way, he kept me in recovery when I wanted to stray from it. I knew that, in order to write, I would have to take my meds. Because, when I hit my rock bottom, I can't write at all. What gave me the drive to write again, to submit for publication, were all these Daniel Craig (in looks only) acting inspired characters dancing around in my head. I started with *Gemini's War*, which was then titled *You Know My Name*.

When I started the blog, it was May 2013. I was published and had twenty-four contracts, or books, total at that. The number of actual books I had published were twenty-four. In October 2019, that number rose to twenty-seven.

I am fond of saying that Maurice Benard got me into treatment, and Daniel Craig kept me there. My love for his body of work is pretty solid. There are the misfires, *Quantum of Solace* and *Spectre*, those are less to do with his performance than with the scripts and directors' mishandling of them. *Spectre* is passable for most of the film, but you can tell that *Quantum of Solace* was written during the writer's strike.

But I digress. The first manuscript I wrote with him as the hero was *Another Way to Die*. It was also the first time a legitimate publisher accepted it. In fact, I had submitted it four publishers, and all of them presented me with a contract. That was a great feeling. I went with MuseItUP Publishing because they develop their writers.

And, let me tell you, my first encounter with an editor was a painful one. It was like having my skin ripped off. I must have cussed her out one hundred different ways to Sunday, but Leah Schizas is an amazing editor. I cussed her because it hurt. But, ultimately, it was a great idea, and a good manuscript became a great book under her edits. It was a steep learning curve, but she was amazing. She is good part of why I'm the writer that I am today, forever grateful, and still learning. But my writing wouldn't be half as good as it is now. I know, however, that I will always be honing my craft, trying to make it to the next level.

I first discovered Daniel Craig in *Casino Royale*, on DVD,

in 2009. In 2010, I wrote *Another Way to Die* during MayNo-WriMo as a part of Coyote Con, a free online writer's convention. And MayNoWriMo was a writing contest where you had to write a 50,000 word book in thirty days.

Daniel was the hero. A black ops, a nefarious organization, in both Gemini's (the heroine) and his pasts tied them together. I enjoyed writing that book immensely. No pressure, no strings, no reason to let up. Writing is addictive. If you are driven to create, then you know what I'm talking about.

If you have bipolar disorder, then you have these wonderful windows of outrageous productivity levels. People will marvel and say, "How did you do that?" It's been my experience they hate us for it, too.

As continued to write from 2011-2013, I had accrued four print books and, whenever I went to Fandom Fest, I sold in only double digits. Not a lot of authors excelled there. To be honest, at a comic con, people do a lot of looking. Then, on the last day, they come back in the hope that authors will offer their books at discount prices, so that they can get rid of their excess inventory.

All my books at the 2013 Fandom Fest featured Daniel as either the model for the hero, or as the titular audience for my memoirs. I sold thirty-four books thanks to my Daniel Craig-inspired mojo. As winter rolled around, my mind began to wonder, *What about a documentary?* I had it in my head about how I wanted it to be, but I couldn't bring myself to pull the trigger on it, that is, until Imaginarium was announced. They included in the announcement that there would also be a small festival.

I quickly messaged Stephen about it. I asked if there would be a documentary category, and he said, "Yes, you should enter your film." (Remember, no actual film existed at that point.) I asked if I could have a Q&A, and a book signing, afterwards. He said, "Yes." That was in February of 2014. Again, no film had yet existed. I had never shot a documentary. And could not, for the life of me, get anyone to sit down and talk openly about bipolar disorder. I had no credibility at that point, only some faint yearning of what once was a powerful dream, to be a Hollywood screenwriter and filmmaker. I had given up all hope of ever going to Hollywood. I figured that my destiny lay in being an author. But, whenever I tried to break through to New York, the answer was always the same. I had a few near misses, including an agent telling me that my story was worthy, but it wasn't right for her. She recommended a male agent, and he wanted nothing to do with me; a form rejection. That was for *The Guardian*, which I'm self-publishing as soon as I get the formatted manuscripts from Stephen Zimmer.

But, back to *Letters to Daniel*. The documentary was very basic. I collected twelve letters from the book, a so-called greatest hits, that strung together a narrative for the audience to follow. I collected photographs and put together a slide show of sorts. No one would sit down with me, so I told my own story. I knew zero voice actresses. At that point, I knew no actresses who were good enough to read my life story. Now, I'm a shitty actress. I really have no business doing it, but I chose to do it myself when no one appeared.

By the end of April, I had finished the documentary for a whopping $345.00, and a lot of help. Bertena Varney assisted me securing a sound studio. Pamela Turner let me edit on her computer, and Danny Jones Jr. gave me his song, "The Wind Blows Through My Garden" to use over the end credits.

I thought that I would screen the finished film at Imaginarium, but it faded away to nothing after that. I imagined it being relegated to a dusty bin, sealed off like so much toxic waste. Not everyone gets the power of that little documentary.

It ended up screening at five festivals, winning five awards along the way. While the premiere garnered me my largest audience for the film, my most triumphant screening would be at AOF Megafest in 2016. Winning Best Social Commentary and the Louis Mitchell Award for Best Feature or Short at such a large festival-in California, no less, was a heady experience. But the first award we ever received for it was at the Indie Gathering. We didn't screen, but won an Honorable Mention there. I entered it on something of a whim. We had four screenplays submitted, and I took a gamble that they would like it.

The goal of any film is for people to see it. And the microfilm and the trailer we submitted would 2nd Place and 3rd Place respectively. But the importance of Indie Gathering's impact on *Letters to Daniel* cannot be overstated. Since 2014, we've been pushing to the *Letters to Daniel* narrative, whether it in book form, documentary, or short form to keep people talking.

The worst was enduring the laughter from some ass when *Letters to Daniel: Awareness* screened, and the end credits song was a little long. My heart nearly exploded out of my chest, and that was just the microfilm.

At AOF, when the logo for our film company came up on screen, the large audience applauded loudly. They clapped again at the end when my name came up on the screen; that was an incredible feeling.

The panic was so bad at Indie Gathering that I couldn't stay for the Q&A. I was embarrassed, and I couldn't face that faction of the crowd who had laughed. I could have handled it if the film wasn't about me, but it was about me, and it felt like they were laughing at me. When it was the film that they were laughing at, that still doesn't make me feel any better.

But the dream persisted. We wrote the narrative screenplay and entered it in several film festivals. It did exceeding well. At

AOF, it never cracked the top scripts, but it always was an official selection, and it had the full support of the festival creator, and the director.

Theresa Weston told me that it deserved to be made into a feature film. Del spent several phone calls, and conversations online, mentoring me. He was always there when I had a question. The dream started to pound in my head.

Like a double-edged sword, I wanted Daniel Craig to see this movie and know, first-hand, how his career has affected mine, and how it has impacted my recovery, because my writing and my recovery are entwined knotted up together. You can't have one without the other.

It's crazy to dream of something like that because, even though when I travel to outside festivals, they know about *Letters to Daniel*, and that's awesome. I know it's on Hollywood's radar, because two SAG actresses were attached to it, only to have to bow out because we weren't below the radar.

I've created an expectation of a product, some hype. I've done it by building a solid brand over the course of six years. This film may not put us on the map, but it may open some closed doors that will allow us to soar into the mainstream. I believe in this film and, hopefully, others will, too.

MY PERSONAL MISSION

*W*hen the *Letters to Daniel* blog was born, I couldn't have foreseen the path that it would take. I loved writing my memoirs because I thought no one would be "listening," as it were. Boy, was I wrong. With little to no effort, the blog simply took off. Being the person that I am, I went to the blog, almost daily, and posted my story and gave an account of what it was like to live with a bipolar disorder diagnosis, and why I was so grateful to be where I was at.

What happened was unexpected, people started reaching out to me, saying that their mother/father/sister/brother, husband/wife had bipolar disorder. The most touching experiences being the ones who told me that they, too, had bipolar and that they saw themselves in my story.

Becoming a mental health advocate was never in the game plan but, with the creation of the *Letters to Daniel* blog, I not only made a way for me to heal, but a way for others like me to feel heard, to feel like they mattered.

I know, in the beginning, when I was first diagnosed, I wanted to create projects whose themes would cover mental illness, and mental health awareness. What I didn't realize was that I was too close to it, raw with the reality of the situation. How could I help anyone else when I couldn't even help myself? How could I write and execute stories about people struggling with, and making peace, with their mental health issues when I had yet to regain some sort of recovery and stability?

The blog changed all that for me. It opened up worlds of possibility. It made me realize that the characters I had created over the years were probably as mixed up and screwed up as me. I had just never identified them as having a mental illness.

I began to incorporate those themes consciously into my work. When I collected the letters into a book, I had no idea that I would take another step down the advocacy road. At conventions, the book led to conversations as to how it had helped them not feel so alone, or how it had helped up them understand their loved one, or even themselves.

I would give the book away if someone had bipolar disorder and couldn't afford it. I also would comfort people who were struggling.

The making of the documentary was another thing altogether. The moment that really set firmly on the advocacy was an interview I did for Del Weston's Action On Film. He told me that I was more than filmmaker, that I was an advocate. It had been something I had been feeling, but not articulating.

I began putting intention behind my documentaries and scripts. Mental health wasn't always the theme, but my experiences better informed my writing choices. My documentaries reflected the different dynamics of bipolar disorder in my family, and what *Letters to Daniel* has meant to my recovery.

Which has led to whole new career as a teacher of the "Thriving Creatively in the Industry While Coping with Serious Mental Illness" seminar/workshop. To say that I have been blessed is really an understatement. To say giving back is just as, if not more, fulfilling than your success doesn't quite do it justice, either.

Since 2016, it has been my dream to travel to college campuses and screen my film and speak to my experiences, and sell my books, to reach out to that marginalized population that has been shunned, and stigmatized, by society and let it know that I was one of them, that speaking their truth out can only heal them.

That, yes, stigma would always be around but that the more of us who stand up and tell our stories, the less that stigma would be. It's my personal mission to stamp out stigma.

As I've related before, I have faced it in many forms. I've been discriminated against at work because of my illness. I've also been ostracized because of it. Some people even see me as looking to beat a dead horse with my advocacy, like I've heard her did this particular song and dance before.

What those people don't realize is they are exactly the reason why my story bears repeating. And, not just my story, but millions of others like mine.

Mental illness is pervasive, and is at epidemic levels. One in five people will experience mental illness during their lifetime. And, if you don't have it, then chances are your life will be touched by it when a loved one does.

The story of *Letters to Daniel* is important to me because it's not just my story, but my caregiver's story as well. When the movie fell apart on multiple occasions, and I despaired it ever getting made, I soldiered on.

Though, quite honestly, the first time it fell through, I was devastated, and I just wanted to lie down and die. I wanted to be done with the film and walk away from it. All the delays over the next four years yielded us a better cast. The only holdovers from the initial cast being Vanessa Card, and Maria Christian. Both of them executed their roles wonderfully. Everyone else fell away when we tried putting the film together.

Not everyone shared our vision. To be fair, a few local people shared our vision. But, on the flip-side, we had tremendous support from those who did. (Stephen Zimmer, Holly Marie Phillipe, Tony Acree, the lovely ladies who showed up to be extras, Marian Allen, and Per Bastet) there were others, people, like Mysti Parker, who allowed us to use her house, as well as other pockets of support.

But *Letters to Daniel* has turned into something special. What started out as a glimmer of a dream had really blossomed. I only wish that I could share the beautiful work performed by my cast and crew in these pages. All I can say is be on the lookout for the film. Hopefully, the avenues of distribution which have presented themselves will open up, and I'll have beautiful memories to share.

My mission is to share my journey so that others may not suffer. My mission is to share my journey so that others might learn about the illness, and know how to treat someone who is struggling, whether it be the person with the illness, or the caregiver.

I think, for people who know me and Missy, that this will be something of a revelation, not about me. Although, they may think less of me for treating Missy so poorly, but my mission is also bringing Missy into the forefront.

We talk about our friendship being like that of Bette Midler, and Barbara Hershey, in *Beaches*. She is forever saying, "I don't want to die like that, from an unknown disease, in shadows, and completely forgotten. And cheated on by a loser husband."

Missy thinks the perception of her is that she is a person who helps me carry my books, and little else, at Imaginarium. I think that people look past Missy, sometimes, because she is quiet and reserved.

One of our friends said, "I want to see Missy do a belly laugh." They wanted to see Missy cut loose and feel things on an intense, and a big, level. Just because she's not demonstrative does not mean Missy doesn't mean Missy doesn't feel things deeply.

Would I say I have bigger emotions? Well, yeah; I have a mood disorder that makes me more sensitive to the goings on around me. Missy just holds her emotions close to the vest.

I guess part of my mission is to show the world just how great Missy is when, most of the time, she resides there in my shadow to some degree.

I want to make the world a better place. Right now, the world is a scary place for anyone who isn't a perceived normie. Read: straight white males, with money, even though the shootings are perpetrated by hate filled, isolated white men.

The irony is not lost on me. I'm all for gun control. I know that's not a popular notion in the South, but there are just some folks who have no business owning a weapon. I include myself in that sentiment.

But, something that I want everyone to know, is what I think about this: 99.9999% of those of us with serious mental illness have no intention of harming another human being, let alone go on a shooting spree ending in tragedy. Most of us are more likely to hurt ourselves rather than anyone else.

Angry and isolated men kill. Sometimes, they are mentally ill, but rarely do the two things intersect.

A majority of those with mental illness are just quietly trying to live our lives, and find a purpose-driven life. That's what I want people to know about those with bipolar disorder. That we're mothers, fathers, husbands, wives, children, siblings, not some stereotype to be used as a political punching bag, and scapegoat for society's ills.

When I see leaders doing that, I wonder if they remember society's history. I feel like our nation is on fire, and it's burning to the ground while Nero fiddles away.

I want *Letters to Daniel* to be a gateway to a larger discussion, and to act as a call to action on everyone's part. These are dangerous times we live in if you're different from the mainstream.

I encourage everyone to research their senators and, if they're trash, like Moscow Mitch McConnell, then I encourage you to vote them out. It is the GOP that stripped Obamacare of mental health parity, among other things.

Sorry for getting political, but these things have affected my treatment, and my ability to properly access it. It's part of what drives me to get out and advocate. If I don't, then who will?

For some, it's as simple as putting a face on it. For others, you can put a million faces on it, and they don't care. Politicians are the worst. I have very definitive views on this. I see a political party rolling back women's rights, human rights, and destroying what this country is supposed to be about.

Since I depend on disability, and the good graces of my parents to survive, (and 90% of those who have bipolar disorder are permanently disabled) *Letters to Daniel* is my way of calling attention to how modern medicine, and the support of friends and family and, yes, government services, when used for the power of good, can, indeed, work miracles.

To bring it into focus, I brought all my talents and those talents of my cast and crew, along with joint leadership with Missy, to bear upon *Letters to Daniel* so that it could be not only a springboard for my and Missy's careers, but a force for good in this world in a time when such a thing is desperately needed.

DEL AND THERESA: PART TWO

*D*el is really a larger than life character. Bold, brash, and unapologetic, he is what he is. A creator, a humanitarian, simply put a force of nature. Theresa is his wife, and partner in all things, with a spine of steel, and a heart of gold. Well, both of them have a heart of gold. Are they protective of their brand that they've worked to build over the last sixteen years? Yes, and that's perfectly understandable. But they also are generous with their time, and their knowledge, not to mention their love.

What they have created is an incubator of creativity. They set up networking events, seminars, screenings, where the point is to mix and mingle with your fellow screenwriters, and filmmakers, to make little AOF babies. (I heard Del say that one time.) The AOF babies being films made by AOFers who have decided to collaborate.

It was at AOF in 2016 where I found two of my greatest assets to *Letters to Daniel*. I like to call us the AOF Southern Connection. Kentucky, me. West Virginia, Clint. Arkansas,

Mark. These gentlemen are not only geniuses in the truest sense of the word, they are gentlemen, too.

Del and Theresa made it possible for me to meet, then build relationships with those two men. Del is a cracker jack, but he loves big. He is always willing to listen, and is always ready with advice.

During 2016, I was a bit of a mess. Traveling to Monrovia, CA cross country with me, and Aunt Sue was something of learning experience, such as, I never want to ride six days in the car with her again. Some of her words of wisdom were cool. But, other than that, she thinks she's been cured of her bipolar disorder. Given that I was going out to California to share my experiences through film on the subject, I really didn't want her chattering on in the background about not using medication.

I think I've made my point of view clear on this, a bipolar individual needs their medication. To go without it can only lead to trouble for that person. To encourage them to go without their medication is not only misguided, but it's also highly irresponsible. Mania, and hypomania, are highly destructive. Depression, potentially fatal. And, when you encourage individuals to go off their medications, you invite disaster and tragedy.

Point being, I was glad to finally be out of that car.

At that first AOF, I really didn't know what to expect. I spied Del putting up the drop banner up, and he noticed me and gave me a big hug and greeted me warmly. To be honest, I was overwhelmed. I didn't know anybody. I was as far away from home as I'd ever been without a buddy, or partner in crime.

People informed me that there were bigger festivals by far. I could only take their word for it. AOF was, and remains to be, the biggest festival that I attend on a yearly basis. I met Susana

Campos, and Christine Whalen, that year, as they were the ones who would come pick me up from the hotel and take me to the Krikorian.

That first year was special in a lot ways. The Creator's Brunch was more intimate. Everyone got a chance to talk about themselves, and their projects. Subsequent brunches were just as awesome, with a lot more people.

The Writer's Gathering is awesome because they have a poetry slam. Rebekah wanted to win it two years in a row. She made a real splash her first year.

There was the Children's Paint and Play Charity Event, where Theresa reached out and said, "Amy, why not come with us?" I did, and it was an amazing time, although I felt awkard.

But what I learned about myself was that I could force myself out of my box. It wasn't easy, though; I clung to the mezzanine and didn't see too many movies. I did suffer a severe panic attack when I thought that my film wouldn't screen. I dissolved into, and an older lady named Sue comforted me and got me through.

I will never forget that kindness I was alone and felt abandoned by those whom I knew who were also there. He was off chasing a woman who wasn't interested in his games. The guy is nice, just a little dysfunctional. But, when he saw my documentary *Letters to Daniel: Breakdown to Bestseller*, he broke down in tears.

When people cry at my films, I find it odd, but comforting. I can't imagine people crying for me because it's never been my experience that people, at least not many of them, cry out of empathy for me.

But, at AOF, I was interviewed by Del. I watched how he handled the actor from the film, and he had him on his toes. Turns out, it was for the movie *Condo Hell*, Amy Wade's movie. AOF Rising Star 2019, bipolar sibling and roommate ate AOF for 2019. Every movie has a behind the scenes story to it. As beautiful as my experience with *Letters to Daniel* was, when I had finally filmed it, Amy had a doozy of a story, herself.

When I finally sat down for my interview, Del was the opposite of the crack jack, flippant, hard charging, and sarcastically funny host he had been before me. He was soft, inquisitive, and supportive, asking perfect questions of about my little proof of concept film.

When I told him that I felt like I didn't belong there, he said, "You're here, aren't you?"

Del and Theresa have watched me grow as a filmmaker, and a writer, over the three years, and four festivals, I'd attended there. And, this year, they awarded with the Most Likely to Be Produced award for my Gemini Rising script, Most Improved Writer and, for film, they gave me the Founder's Award for my body of work.

What's the Founder's Award? They have been watching me progress, knowing that I have certain challenges that others might not face. Even so, the award, itself, is beautiful, but it also entails something else.

I was awarded a festival that seeks to serve the mentally ill artist who is healing themselves through their art. What a magnificent mission to have for a film festival. I want an advocacy legacy, and what a way to give back! To give other individuals like me the kind of opportunity AOF has given me. I look forward to watching filmmakers, and screenwriters, develop as Del and Theresa have watched me do so.

Could I have foreseen all this that first year?

Wished for it, maybe, but foreseen it? No. But Del has a gift or getting the best from his creators. He gives them the chance to make their careers happen. He sees things in you that maybe you don't see in yourself, or maybe you've lost sight.

That first year at AOF, I was a bit of a wounded bird. *Letters to Daniel* had fallen apart, I had gotten entangled to two bad situations where representation is concerned and was involved with another bad situation (I just didn't know it). I went to AOF looking to make the most of the California experience. I hoped to make connections. I wasn't worried about *Letters to Daniel* because I had been lied to about the fact that we needed 20K for the film.

I was just there to experience the festival and meet people and see my movie. I had zero expectations of winning. To be honored for your work at a competitive festival is a heady experience.

AOF draws world class screenwriting and filmmaking talent. To find yourself among the nominees is the real win. To actually win is just the icing on the cake. When Missy and I won for Best New Writer at AOF, it was a watershed moment. It was a large festival, where the talent we were nominated against was incredible. To triumph with my friends, Andrew and James, in attendance, was wonderful.

Del and Theresa have a way of nurturing you and driving you to continue to excel by showering you with this unconditional love. To put it bluntly, we know a man who has a misfit army doing his bidding, but he manipulates and tears them down.

Del and Theresa have a misfit family, only Del is in the business of building up his filmmakers, and screenwriters, providing them with the knowledge, and connections, to make their dreams come true.

Not every festival can say they do that, Indie Gathering changes lives in that it allows you to connect with other filmmakers, actors, etc., to build your cast and crew. My presence at Indie Gathering allowed me a presence, and a following, in Ohio where a majority of the cast came from.

AOF gives you the power to make your play for the mainstream Hollywood studio system. Indie Gathering has their success stories, too.

Ray Szuch, and Kristina, have the same family vibe with a relaxed, laid back atmosphere. They network, but a weekend pass pre-walk up is $45.00 dollars. Each entry gets you a VIP badge, whether you win, are selected, or not. Walk up is $55.00, and their overall championship belts are the coolest thing this side of the Mason Dixon.

These places are the highlight of my year of traveling. There is a really cool vibe that allows for each of them to mean different things to me. Indie Gathering has a screenwriting competition that draws just as much talent as AOF.

At AOF, Theresa is like that mother hen who is making sure the show goes off without a hitch and that her screenwriters and filmmakers are cared for. The only way to really run afoul of Del is to make Theresa unhappy, or to hurt his family. I wonder why people insist on doing this. First of all, Del's family is beautiful. Second, it's just bad business, and you shouldn't be surprised when he reacts adversely.

Kristina is a lot like Del in that she can remember what project is from what person. Even if you have multiple projects, she's on it.

Indie Gathering is where to go to get started. Their goal is turn screenwriters into filmmakers, either as directors, producers, or both.

AOF seeks to show you how dream impossibly big. Del once called me a termite, meaning that I'm always working. I believe that there are people who will always do better than you but, conversely, there will always be people who aren't as fortunate as you. Del and Theresa, and Ray and Kristina, are very much all about keeping your eyes on your own lane.

I'm very much of the belief if you work hard, and place yourself in the position of having success and celebrate each step along the way, then you will get there.

LEA SCHIZAS & MUSEITUP, FRANK HALL & HYDRA, DAVE MATTINGLY & BLACKWYM

In the beginning, it was all about being a published author, both for me and Missy. Breaking through to New York was all I ever dreamed about for a long time as a kid. Some people are fortunate enough in their late teens, and early twenties, to attend college. As they grow older, they attend workshops, and seminars, which expand their knowledge and skill of their chosen trade or career.

I attended Eastern New Mexico University in Portales, NM. I chose to major in theater arts. It was a lousy fit. The class I really excelled at was the film studies class where we watched, and discussed, films of all types.

And, in college, my illness stuck me pretty hard, so it led to me dropping out. I used to say, "I want to go back." Now, all I feel is choking sense of anxiety when I think about going back to get my degree.

As I watched films, I was able to learn a lot but, mostly, I wrote every day during my early twenties. When I was sick, and wandering aimlessly through the bipolar desert the dream of writing loomed large like an oasis I couldn't quite reach.

As I said, in 2010 I wrote, *Another Way to Die*. That was in May. Toward the end of the year, Missy's dad remained in the hospital, due to complications from liver transplant surgery, and I was left at home a lot to hold down the fort, as it were.

As I typed up a script I had written, and edited *Another Way to Die*, I became increasingly aware of the fact that my career wasn't just going to magically happen. In other words, the mountain wasn't going to come me. I was going to have to go to the publishing mountain.

Pamela Turner was having some success on the digital forefront with her book *Deathsword*, (excellent novel, by the way. You should check it out, as well as her other books) so I decided that I would submit *Another Way to Die* to Lyrical Press. (Lyrical is now a part of Kensington, which is New York traditional publisher, so bravo on that front Pam) For the first time, I didn't get a straight-out rejection, I got a revise and resubmit.

I must say that I had no idea what I needed to do in order to fit my manuscript to their mission statement, but I sure as hell tried and, then, I resubmitted. In the interim, Pam told me about Digicon, a free online writer's conference about self-publishing, and electronic publishing. Savvy Authors was putting it on, and she highly recommended it.

This was exactly the opportunity I needed. At the time, Missy and I were sharing an apartment and getting out and enjoying the simplest of things was hard to do. Neither of us were flush with cash, so it was the simple things that we enjoyed: Starbucks, Barnes and Noble, the movies. And, when we went to the movies, there was no popcorn, no so soda, nor red vines, no nothing.

So, after dinner during the evenings, I attended workshops,

seminars, and I pitched to small press publishers. I can't remember all their names, but each of them either offered me a contract, or asked me for the full manuscript.

As I stated earlier, I signed with MuseItUp Publishing. It would prove to be a beneficial relationship. I contracted for seven books, and five saw publication. The nice thing about small presses is that you receive individual attention, whereas, there is more of a chance that you would get lost in the shuffle at bigger houses. Lea Schizas is passionate when it comes to Muse-ItUP, and its various imprints. And her authors, editors, and cover artists are an extension of her own family.

When I signed with Muse, it was the first time that I felt validated as a writer. I had fallen into the trap of sham, and vanity presses, before; what confirmed to me that Muse was not a vanity press was when I received the covers for *Another Way to Die* and *No Ordinary Love*. They were gorgeous, and totally professional (artist, Delilah Stephans) looking.

I was excited, to say the least. With a January 2012, release date I was ready to go. (It was only February of 2011.) In April, I wrote a sci-fi erotica piece called *No Ordinary Love*, which was quickly snatched up for publication and given an October 2011 release date. In the following months, I would correspond with my editors a sweet woman from Malta, and my line editor, Greta Gunselman. I became friendly with Lea as well.

Muse was a good, healthy, nurturing place for me to blossom during my early writing career, so much so that Lea planted the seed for what would become *Letters to Daniel* and, ultimately, that influenced my transformation into a mental health advocate.

I would do NaNoWriMo in November of 2011, inspired by a Harlequin Love Inspired historical about a Roman soldier and woman headed for certain death, (it was set in the past and a little puritanical for my tastes) music from the *Gladiator* sound-track/score, and a blurb about a dystopian YA book, I sat down and conceived *The Gladiator Chronicles*. It was an absolute blast writing it, as well as imagining a buff Daniel Craig as a tortured gladiator forced to choose: do the evil queen's bidding, or risk certain death by serving another.

It was the trilogy, but I only ever wrote the first two books. The first complete trilogy I wrote the first book is out from Three Bitches Press. Those two books would eventually be put together and released as a print book. But my first print book would come from Frank Hall, who, at the time was the owner, and publisher, of Hydra Publications, a local press located in Madison, Indiana.

I was doing a signing at his then store and was telling him about the book I had written, and that I really wanted a print deal. He told me to send it to him.

Well, I went home and immediately shot it off to him. He sent me back a contract. I love Frank, he battles heavily with depression, but he did a beautiful with that publishing house. He gave a lot of local writers a home, a chance to be heard, a chance to have their work read by the world, a chance to hold their work in their hot, little hands.

I attended my first convention with an actual book to sell at Conglomeration. During those early days, Tony Acree and Rachel Rawlings met at Olive Garden on Outer Loop. It's hard to believe that was six, or seven, years ago. At that first Conglomeration, Tony showed what a slick salesman he was. He was a blast to be around.

Marian Allen was a sweetie, too, a supporter of *Letters to Daniel*, she had titles published with Hydra, as did Rachel Rawlings. We were like the anti-four horsemen of the apocalypse. We took our meals together and Conglomeration handed out sodas, and waters, to keep us all hydrated.

Conglomeration was the second place I ever sat on panels, a place where the crowds were smaller, and less intimidating. The reality is there are several cons in Kentucky, just not very many that have any true place for authors. They're basically autographs, playing games, and cosplaying, and cosplayers are notoriously tightfisted. That's not a criticism, just a statement of fact.

But, at that first Conglomeration, I remember selling copies and trying to keep up with Tony, but I don't know if anyone can really keep up with Tony. What was great was that I was used to being exposed to University of Louisville fans, except for when I was with Missy, and Tony was and is a University of Kentucky fan. If it wasn't for Frank, none of that would have been possible. Eventually, he sold Hydra to Tony, and Tony began to build his own little publishing empire locally. *Bounty Hunter* was my first print book, and I couldn't be prouder that it was published with Hydra Publications.

Finally, when I had a bad experience with a publishing house, and had to return my advance, I stumbled upon Blackwyrm Publications, and Dave Mattingly. I had found the perfect home for *You Know My Name*. Dave didn't like the title, and I knew, as big publishers were wanting to do, he did a renaming by committee. I didn't care for that. But he understood that my book was, at its heart, a love story, albeit a really fucked up love story, surrounded by shadow groups, and action/adventure.

It was for a trilogy, the name for those three books was *Gemini Rising*. The three volumes were to be named *Gemini's War*, *Gemini's Legacy*, and *Avenging Gemini*. Only two of the titles would be published.

The first one, *Gemini's War*, would go on to be a Top Ten

Amazon Bestseller. Dave was, and is, a really sweet guy, but running a publishing house is a labor-intensive endeavor, and his contracts weren't the clearest things ever written.

His business partner took advantage of that and robbed him blind, crippling the company. Then, there were some personal crises on the home front that just made it impossible for the company, as it was, to go on.

Frank had left the company's titles on Amazon while he figured out what to do with his business, and Dave took them down and reverted the rights back to the authors.

The sum total of the point of this chapter is to show that I had some amazing people whom I had the good fortune of coming into contact with. They all impacted my writing, for the better, by assigning me editors who knew what they were doing. They refined my voice, taught me story structure, and gave me a clue about character development. And, in some cases, I have formed longtime friendships with them which have enriched my life.

MuseItUP is an e-publisher up in Canada. And Hydra Publications (and its various imprints) is now located in LaGrange, KY, USA. And, if you have manuscript you think is ready for publication, those are two of the most reputable places I can think to share it with.

39

TURNING YOUR BIGGEST WEAKNESS
INTO YOUR SHARPEST SWORD

*H*ow? I guess that's the biggest question. If I'm honest, I've always been unable to put on airs, or be someone I'm not. To some, that's refreshing yet, to a lot of people, that is a very threatening thing. If you can be your most authentic self, in other words, embracing who, and, what, you are, then no one can stop you. That's the big secret.

For me, it happened in stages. I've always been an oddball, a weirdo, an other, as the show, *Lost*, put it. I never cared about what other people thought of me, at least not enough to twist myself into something that I wasn't, even when I would screw up in a major way, (like the time I was on stage in a trivia contest and tried to change my answer post fact). And, believe me, I paid for it. People hated me, and they delighted in my failure (I was twelve, people, let it go).

I spent a good deal of my adolescence in emotional pain. High school was way better, but kids are cruel and, when they smell blood, they can be merciless.

So what does any of this have to do with the making of

Letters to Daniel? During my junior year in high school, I began to struggle. Yes, in my life I have faced many ugly things: bullies, abuse, the wicked side of bipolar disorder, even poverty, and hunger. But, at sixteen, my mind began to betray me.

In college, I couldn't fall asleep, which precipitated me missing morning classes. I felt odd, uncomfortable in my own skin, like the world was passing me by. I was hopelessly out of sync, and my inability to connect with others was exaggerated by my not knowing anyone on campus.

My first semester there was hell. I mean, my roommate was nice enough, and I loved being on the debate team. I was half in love with my debating partner, Michael Sifuentes. I enjoyed the college bowl, where we cleaned everyone's clock, including those sufferable fraternity teams who thought they were the shit.

But, other than those few bright spots, my first semester was a bust. Depression quickly set in, as did the homesickness and insomnia. It's hard to function when your mind is beset with booby traps to stymie you. Credit to Mom, she knew that something was wrong but, being over 1,000 miles away from me, she could set the counseling appointments up, but she could not make me keep them.

You see, I didn't want to believe that something was wrong with me. I was just having trouble sleeping, I was just coping with stress. I didn't even occur to me that a time bomb had been ticking away inside my head, waiting for the right mix of ingredients to ignite it. I really had no idea what was going on with me.

I just knew that my classes were impossible to make, that mingling with people wasn't something I wanted to do. Inside, it felt like I was dying a thousand deaths. I was in complete free fall, grasping at the emptiness, and struggling to hold on.

The second semester, I made two friends, and there was a guy who kissed me. It didn't go anywhere. He was too normal, I think. The second guy I was attracted to was just as dysfunctional as me. My freak flag flew way out of control and, a week after meeting me, he said, "I love you." HUGE red flag in retrospect.

Billy had his issues: an abusive father, a controlling mother. And I ran headlong into that, without looking back. I was upset with my family. I hadn't been talking to them until about a week before I left. I disagreed, a great deal, with them about the pressures that they placed me under.

Mom always thought that I was rebelling by getting bad grades. In my family, anything lower than an A is unacceptable. With my brain misfiring, I was unable to live up to theirs, and my, high expectations. My grades suffered. This carried over into my senior year.

Brandy and I weren't close, but she ended up making friends with some of my snootier friends in Neal and Jacob.

When they asked, "Was it really as bad as I said it was?"

Brandy said, "No." It was bad.

And, that summer, it led to a physical altercation between me and my mom.

Mom has chosen to, conveniently, forget that less than stellar moment for either of us. But it's as clear as day to me. Mom is on Zoloft now, and has faced her own mortality ever since. She's a different person now, as am I. I'm not as angry as I used to be, the hurt isn't fresh. Now, the hurts are fewer and farther between.

But, after returning home from college, I was unable to get my shit together for a sophomore year. And, with my brain not doing so well, it wouldn't have mattered if I had managed to get it together.

A few years passed until I got a job at B. Dalton's Book-sellers. I started writing regularly, met Missy, trained for and ran a marathon.

Missy proposed a writing partnership. I said, "Yes."

Life was going good, until it wasn't.

It was the little things at first: the pressurized speech, the dilating pupils, then the inability to finish sentences. My thoughts seemed to trip over one another. Sleep eluded me, bit by bit.

Irritability turned to frustration. I would drive Missy to write twenty-four pages a night with the singular plea of, "One more scene, just one more scene."

Until, finally, I was in pieces emotionally, spiritually, and psychologically, and could no longer write. I could not sleep. I could not eat. At my darkest, I was not even bathing, or brushing my teeth. I was a shell. I mean, I took up space and I was breathing but I was not living. I was not dreaming. I was completely unable to function. It's a terrible place to be because you can't help yourself, let alone help someone understand why you're acting the way that you are.

So how can you make something like that your sharpest weapon to do battle with? First of all, I had to go get evaluated for depression and manic depression, and it would take a few tries. I was diagnosed with manic depression (now called bipolar disorder, for less stigmatizing, purposes) initially, at nineteen. But, instead of embracing the psychiatrist in Artesia, NM, I called a cousin, and she said, "All they want to do is pump you full of pills." That scared me off proper from the psychiatrist, and the medication aspect of it, right away. It would take five years of wondering what was wrong with me.

I know, I had the answer and I had just thrown it away like so much trash, but that has to do with the terrible stigma that is associated with bipolar disorder. I know it's easier in this culture; it's more acceptable for women to reach out for help. And I know that there are intersectional issues, and challenges, that I don't have the first clue about. But how you flip the script is how you embrace your diagnosis and do the hard work of daily recovery.

How do you flip the script? I'll be honest, I had to wander in bipolar desert alone for a long time. Going to the doctor, suffering, healing in inches, the darkness is always there, watching, waiting for its moment to pounce. You have to fight for your recovery. Now, one else can do it for you. Cobble the good days together. Be kind to yourself on the bad days because, with this disease, that's the reality; there will be bad days. But you'll find, as you roam the desert, that there are beautiful things to be found there. As someone with this mood disorder, let me tell you that you will feel, and experience, things on deeper level: colors are more vibrant, love is felt deeper, the scent of perfume is sweeter, and the smell of fresh cut grass can send you tripping back through childhood, and give you all the feelings.

Again, you ask, "How do you go from being lost in the desert to soaring and living your dream?" You do have to do the hard work of recovery. Some days, that will be easier than others. What worked for me was the reawakening of my creative voice, that within the first year of being diagnosed. Purposely writing every day was something I wandered away from, thinking that, for a novel, I would have to always write scripts, and I could write when co-writing. While scripts are always a co-written affair, novels were not. In 2007, I began to write every day four to eight hours a day, depending on if I was writing by hand, or typing on a computer.

I began to go into town with Missy and spend the day at Borders, writing, and drinking coffee. As I did this, I began to discipline myself into writing every day. When I acquired a laptop, writing switched from writing for a certain timeframe to how many words I wrote a day, and I reached for 1,667 words a day.

Then, I added walking to my regime. I kept my appointments with my pdoc, and therapist. I was honest about my emotions, and I learned to take ownership of my actions, using "I" statements.

Finally, I wrote something that the publishers liked. Lea, in early 2012, suggested a bipolar writers' blog. I pushed the suggestion aside. But when May 7, 2013 arrived, and I was halfway through an open fan letter, I decided that blog the idea might work as my memoirs.

What I was doing was journaling and, as I journaled, I got stronger emotionally, and psychologically, until I was beginning to advocate. First, through my book. Then, through my documentary. And, now, finally, my narrative film, and mental health festival, advocating for the mentally ill.

That's how *I* managed to flip the script. And if this bipolar diagnosed girl can do it, then so can you.

40

A FEW CLOSING THOUGHTS &
ADVICE

Letters to Daniel, from blog to finished film, took me six years. Along the way, there were false starts, lies, promises, both kept and unkept, setbacks, and finally a finished film. There were times when I wanted to walk away and give it all up. Making a film is hard to begin with, bringing your passion project to life is even harder. And, when it's your life, it's warts and all, scary as hell.

But it was my dream of dreams, to make a beautiful movie, to feel like a legit, for real filmmaker, not a pretender. I wanted it to launch me and Missy into a life of paid studio gigs screenwriting for others. I want us to be able to leave this state in the rearview. I mean, I love Kentucky; my family is here, I've recovered and built my indie career in part here, but there comes a time where the birdie needs to leave the nest.

I would love to go live in Vegas. I know people there, and we would be close to my dear friends, Andrew and James, who would be only an hour plane ride away.

I guess as hard and as arduous as the journey has been to get

255

Letters to Daniel made, only half of the job is done. Now, we have to seek out distribution, get it to film festivals. But, to me, we did the thing. We did it right and, now, it's time to take it out and show it off.

My thoughts on this, I could have given up at any time. God knows that I got knocked down countless times, shot myself in the foot, got in my own way. But, with the support of Missy, my parents, and the people kind enough to let their homes be a part of my little dream, I feel like I can change the world.

Well, I didn't set out to change anything. This whole process profoundly changed me. It made realize that I am much tougher than I gave myself credit for because, even when the situation was untenable, and I wanted to cry, "Uncle," I would face down my fears, and my critics.

In 2018, after ICFF, I had to go into a darkened room and have a serious talk with myself. Did I absolutely have to direct this script? Was everyone right to doubt me? Del was so wonderful on an open post on Facebook he simply wrote, *"Direct!"*

It wasn't long after I resolved that I was making the film with Missy, and I was going to direct it. I had my dream team. I just demanded to make the film; I started looking for at least an executive producer to help with the raising of money. At Indie Gathering, that door opened for us.

I guess what I want to tell you is that, if you have a dream, then don't wait for someone else's permission to pursue it. We have a finite amount of time on this earth. I realized that I was waiting for the perfect circumstances to exist for me to make *Letters to Daniel.*

I allowed myself to forget the biggest lesson I had learned as an indie and small press author. There will never be a so-called perfect time. You have to screw your courage, up and take that leap of faith.

I can hear the excuses now.

"But I have a family."

Stephen King had a family.

"But, my wife/husband won't let me."

Well, then, you have some serious choices to make. How happy are you going twenty, thirty years down the road, knowing you let your dreams die for the person who kept you from them?

"But I have no money."

It is my experience that people can find the money to do what they love.

What it boils down to is, what are your priorities in life?

I believe that, if you treat something like a hobby in the sense that it's not serious outlet, but something you do only when you "have time," then you're not someone I can relate to.

I love what I do. I don't have time, I make time. You say, "I don't have the time." Well, that's just bullshit. What I'm hearing is that it's not a priority. And, that's okay, just don't tell me that you want it more than anything else in this world because, if that's the case, then you will move Heaven and Earth to make it happen.

Letters to Daniel started out as a seed someone else planted in my creative brain. For years, I wanted to tell my story, and the story just wouldn't come out of me. Sometimes, things have to cook for a while, like stories, and lifelong dreams.

I wanted to make a movie with real film equipment, talented actors, and an experienced crew. My first movie with Missy was a disaster. Our second movie, *Going Under*, was well-acted, but poorly shot. But one of the actors was a skilled graphic artist, and photographer. He made us a wonderful poster for it.

That was in 2004 and 2005. The movies were not technically sound, therefore, they were never seen by the outside world. *Letters to Daniel* marks a departure for us. We went for quality, and we got it. I'm so proud of our cast and crew. I'm so glad that I didn't give up, and that Missy didn't give up on me.

So my advice to you, if you want to make a movie, then make it one you are passionate about creating because it's not only going to be hard, it's going to seem damn near impossible. What's that story that's been burning a hole in your gut?

You think, *but I've never written a story before, let alone pulled a cast and crew together.* Find a partner who either has knowledge of those things, or is willing to learn to do it alongside you. Invest in yourself. There are any number of online classes in production, for both writing and directing. There's the Sundance Collab, Stage32, Script Lab, ScreenwritingU. There are fellowships, such as the Stowe Story Labs, Sundance (one for producers, directors, and writers alike). Executives, producers, and writers, populate social media. Gaining one as a mentor would help your career tremendously.

Another tactic is a screenwriting workshop or seminar given by the likes of Robert McKee, or Michael Hauge. They give you the fundamentals, and the real meat and potatoes, of storytelling structure. I took Michael Hauge's class and read *How to Write A Screenplay in 21 Days*, Syd Field's *Screenplay*, and a myriad of other books about screenwriting, including William Goldman's, *Which Lie Did I Tell: More Adventures in the Screentrade.*

If you're dreaming of writing that Oscar-winning script, the time is now. Or, maybe, you dream of having a show on television. That thing about having no money? It cost very little to write. If you don't have a computer, buy a notebook, and a legal pad. John Grisham wrote his first novel on legal pads. I wrote my first scripts the same way. My first novels I typed on a word processing typewriter after midnight because I worked the third shift at a movie rental store.

Writing is the most blissful part of the movie making process for me. It's stress free, and allows me to venture into any world that I want to and not worry about production value, how I'm going to pull it off in reality. I just channel the characters, and the story will write itself.

That story idea burning a hole in your head? That one keeping you up at night, forcing you to think, *What if?* Well, stop thinking about what if and take the leap.

The way I'm able to write so much so fast, I write one hundred words at time and, if I still feel like going, then I write one hundred more. And so on and so on, you get the point.

Time's a wastin', as they say in these parts. No one is going to write your movie for you, so you might as well get started on it, yourself. There is no greater feeling of accomplishment than the finishing of a project that you are passionate about.

Here's another cold hard fact. The only person who wants to make your passion project as badly as you do, is... you. Hollywood is as risk averse as ever. In a perfect world, your glorious script would be funded, and it would be a beautiful experience when it gets produced.

The reality is that, these days, agents and writers are at odds. And, usually, they don't want to read a whole script; they will want to see what is called a rip reel. I don't have the ability to make these. I mean, I tried, but I'm not very good at it.

Mostly there's the catch-22; they want to see if you've had anything produced and, in order to be produced you often need a manager, or an agent, to unlock those particular doors for you.

I recommend diving in and start honing your filmmaking craft. I directed eleven documentaries, various music videos, short films, micro films, and proof of concept trailers. But I don't have the proper equipment, you say. A lot of festival films are being shot on an iPhone. There are various things to help enhance iPhone films, such as lights and microphones. Amazon is a good place to start. You may have to wade through a lot of crap in order to get to what you need but access, and, good pricing makes them hard to beat.

But, if have a mentor, then they can steer you the stores that the professionals use. They can tell you what equipment is essential. For my first films, I used a small camcorder from Walmart, natural light, and the camera microphone. Now, my films suffered in overall quality for it, but it served me well as a developing director, and filmmaker.

What I am saying is that I made my dream come true with a lot of helping hands, and generous hearts. And the simple fact is that I think you can, too. *Letters to Daniel* is on the verge of a new journey, and me along with it. To say I am ready is an understatement, so bring it on!